Nursing
Mo✔ KT-500-415

To Derek, Gareth and Brendan,
with all my love

For Baillière Tindall

Publisher Jacqueline Curthoys/Alex Mathieson
Project Manager Ewan Halley
Project Development Editor Karen Gilmour
Project Controller Pat Miller/Jane Shanks

Nursing in the new NHS: Modern, Dependable?

Anita Fatchett

MA BA(Hons) RN RHV CertEd RNT
Senior Lecturer in Nursing,
Leeds Metropolitan University, Leeds, UK

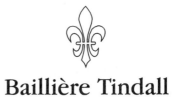

Baillière Tindall

Edinburgh   London   New York   Philadelphia   Sydney   Toronto   1998

BAILLIÈRE TINDALL
An imprint of Harcourt Brace and Company Limited

Baillière Tindall, 24–28 Oval Road, London NW1 7DX, UK
The Curtis Center, Independence Square West, Philadelphia, PA
19106–3399, USA
Harcourt Brace and Company, 55 Horner Avenue, Toronto, Ontario,
M8Z 4X6, Canada
Harcourt Brace and Company, Robert Stevenson House, 1–3 Baxter's
Place, Leith Walk, Edinburgh EH1 3AF, UK
Harcourt Brace and Company – Australia, 30–52 Smidmore Street,
Marrickville, NSW 2204, Australia
Harcourt Brace and Company – Japan, Ichibancho Central Building,
22-1 Ichibancho, Chiyoda-ku, Tokoyo 102, Japan

First published 1998

ISBN 0 7020 2301 9

British Library Cataloguing in Publication Data
A catalogue record for this book is available from the British Library.

Library of Congress Cataloging in Publication Data
A catalog record for this book is available from the Library of
Congress.

Medical knowledge is constantly changing. As new information
becomes available, changes in treatment, procedures, equipment and
the use of drugs become necessary. The editor, contributors and
publishers have, as far as it is possible, taken care to ensure that the
information given in this text is accurate and up to date. However,
readers are strongly advised to confirm that the information,
especially with regard to drug usage, complies with latest legislation
and standards of practice.

Printed by Bell and Bain Ltd, Glasgow

Contents

Preface

The National Health Service ranks as one of the most successful innovations in social policy of the century. It represents a brave assertion of the equal value of human life, by ensuring that patients get the treatment they need, rather than the treatment they can afford. (Cook 1994)

Thanks to the National Health Service (NHS), the population of the UK has largely been entitled to health care free at the point of need for 50 years. The NHS is something of which we can be justifiably proud in the country, reflecting as it does a society expressing a practical concern for the health and well-being of all its members.

The NHS has, of course, accumulated its own fair share of faults, two of which in particular are worthy of mention at this early stage. First, a low priority in practice has been given to the prevention of ill health, with the greatest attention and professional status given to the treatment of illness and hospital care. Second, the glamour and prestige of surgery, high technology and the creation of ever more splendid hospitals have swallowed up a disproportionate amount of health care resources. This has effectively side-lined attention away from the broader, more socially useful primary health care setting, in which the majority of the population experience their health care whether at primary, secondary or tertiary levels.

As the millennium approaches with a new government at the helm, there are many issues which need to be addressed within the NHS – not least, the direction in which the Labour administration intends it to go. After all, the decade of health care reform set in motion by the Thatcher Government of the early 1980s which 'threw' NHS structures and personnel up into the air, has ended in the late 1990s with the Conservative Government out of office, a new Labour Government, and the emergence of the so-called 'Primary care-led National Health Service; (NHSME 1995). The rhetoric of this apparent substantial shift in focus for the NHS is potentially very exciting, as it could open up many new avenues in care for primary health care nurses, together with important health gains for the whole population. However, while the new vision has struck a cord with many, the challenge now is to influence moves beyond the slogan and to ensure the continued contribution of professionally qualified nurses to the developing primary health care setting.

Anita Fatchett 1998

REFERENCES

Cook R 1994 In: Fatchett A. Politics, policy and nursing. Baillière Tindall, London
NHSME (National Health Service Management Executive) 1995 Priorities and planning guidance for the NHS: 1996/97. EL (95) 68. NHSME, Leeds

Acknowledgements

Thank you to Jenny Stronach, Jacqui Parkin, Camille Haigh, Paula Wainwright, Clare Werry and Zeba Siddiq for processing my work.

1

Setting the scene

The National Health Service (NHS) is a much loved institution, ranking second only to the monarchy in the nation's affections. As such, each succeeding incoming government, whether a Conservative or Labour administration, has stated its continued support for the development of a thriving NHS. Therefore it was no surprise that Prime Minister Blair, speaking on behalf of a newly elected Labour Government, referred supportively to the NHS in his opening address to the nation on the steps of 10 Downing Street on Friday 2 May 1997. He said:

A new Labour Government . . . remembers that it was a previous Labour Government that formed and fashioned the Welfare State and the National Health Service. It was our proudest creation. It shall be our job and our duty to modernise it for a modern world.

This statement of intent both reflected the Labour Party's General Election manifesto commitments for a new and changed health service agenda, and pointed towards immediate policy activity to be announced in the Queen's speech at the State Opening of Parliament 12 days later.

As the Queen pronounced:

My Government is committed to the development of the National Health Service, as a service providing care on the basis of need to the whole population. They will bring forward new arrangements for decentralisation and co-operation within the service, and for ending the internal market. A White Paper will be published on measures to reduce tobacco consumption, including legislation to ban tobacco advertising. (14 May 1997, House of Lords)

The change of Government from Conservative to Labour, after 18 years offered the opportunity for a new administration with a different ideological perspective and mission both to halt and to redirect the process of fundamental change and reform within the NHS which had changed both the context and content of health care delivery.

Under four successive Conservative administrations, nurses, midwives and health visitors had felt the impact of major political and managerial change within the NHS whether in hospital or primary health care settings. Increasingly, they had found themselves working within a commercialised and fragmented organisation, feeling the impact of shortages and strict rationing of resources. For many this was not an easy time, particularly for those in face-to-face contact with the patients and users of the service. The specific promise of more power and choice for all had not been matched with the means to meet this idealistic aim, not least against a backcloth of encouragement for raised consumer expectations and demands. In one sense, nurses and other care professionals had found themselves, to coin a phrase, stuck between a rock and a hard place – in many instances, they had been asked to do the impossible with very little in the way of resources and back-up. As a result, professional morale and self-belief had plummeted on many occasions during the 18-year period of Conservative health and welfare reform.

Mixed messages also had clearly helped to obfuscate the situation. On the one hand the National Health Service Management Executive had set out ambitious and positive sounding strategies for nurses throughout the period of reform, reminding them, and others, that: 'improving health and making care services better is heavily dependent upon their contributions' (NHSME 1993). On the other hand, the credibility of all care professionals, including nurses, had been under attack and in doubt. Like many of the disappointed consumers in the reformed health service, nurses also had felt let down as the impact of the ever deepening programme of health care reform and change had relentlessly progressed. The impacts on professional practice and development had been both profound and wide ranging.

The election then of a Labour Government in May 1997, with a health agenda which on the face of it looked more sympathetic in scope, and gentler in ideology than hitherto, potentially offered a new opportunity for both nurses and nursing to regain and to develop some new professional ground. Having said that, while it might be tempting and, for some possibly, cathartic to tear up old roots and to start all over again (if that were possible), this would surely be a counterproductive move. It is important to learn from, and to build upon, our recent experiences.

In spite of many acknowledged difficulties, much progress has been achieved both professionally and organisationally. It is only sensible to hold on to that which is constructive and positive, and to seek to reverse or to remove only those aspects considered antipathetic to professional practice and development, and to the provision of high quality, modern nursing care. Only a professional dinosaur would surely wish in total to return to pre 1979 or even 1948 agendas. Health care delivery and professional nurse practice need to move with the times and to respond to the changing environment of health needs. It is also already evident that we will only gain the right to develop professionally under this government, or any government, if we take on the responsibility of coordinating appropriate and modern professional nurse responses to the needs of the complex health agendas.

To do this nurses need to develop a broader understanding of the combinations of forces which have led to the situation in which they now find themselves. Indeed, a failure to understand and to learn from recent history could well result in a failure to survive as a profession. Admittedly this particular challenge will not be an easy one to achieve. While the health agenda of the new and differently focused administration has apparently offered a gentler, less competitive, more health-focused programme, it has not offered the promise of an easy ride for anyone – public or professional alike. The striving for financial efficiency, and the search for the proof of the effectiveness of care delivery in every area of the health service will continue, as will the requirement for all professionals of whichever discipline to prove the value of their expert professional contribution. The right to claim such a status, and all that this implies, will only be given to those who are prepared to take up the heavy responsibility for the continued development of both their knowledge and skills well beyond that of initial qualification and appointment to practice.

There is a need to break out of the now increasingly outdated straitjacket of traditional nurse disciplines, and to look towards the creation of more relevant professional roles, offering new and different combinations of skills and knowledge, combined with the ability to offer flexibility and creativity in care, appropriate to, and focused upon assessed local needs and circumstances. This will require ever greater individual responsibility for life-long learning, an ability to reflect on practice and to the development of new ways of working. It will involve the carrying out and the use of research, an increased understanding of, and influence upon health policy making, together with the ability to manage change both for oneself and for others. Importantly, the adaptation to new ways of working as a professional nurse will rely upon the ability to work effectively and in close collaboration with many other disciplines across the developing primary health care settings. Those who merely rest on their laurels gained in earlier times may well lose much of their present role to others, and with this the opportunity for work enrichment and satisfaction as professional nurses in the future.

This book will aim to consider these important issues in greater detail. In Chapters 2–8 the discussions will try to help nurses to clarify what appears to have been going on around them in recent years. Consideration will be given to the historical background and political reasoning behind the changes and the issues which are now in the political ascendancy. The author will examine all of these from a nurse's point of view.

As we will see the NHS reforms were just one part of the wider political plans and ideological raison d'être of the previous Conservative Governments.

Their welfare reforms involved financial retrenchment and tightening up of spending in all areas of health and social care delivery. The effects of these moves not only had an impact on the wider contextual setting of nurse caring, but inevitably, their knock-on effects have made an impression over time on the content of that care. In these ways it will be argued that outside political forces appeared to have been controlling and shaping developments within and around the nursing profession. The outcome of this has not necessarily, it will be suggested, always been for the better.

In a previous discussion of the impact of health service reforms (Fatchett 1994), it was argued that there was a need to develop a will to create strategies to redirect our futures for ourselves, and to avoid being pushed into a shape created by others who appeared neither to support the NHS, nor understand the role of nurses. However, now that there is a Labour Government which appears to be offering a changed and more supportive vision for both an NHS and a nursing profession, we cannot just sit back and assume a rosy future. We need to take part in, and to influence the political debates around health care, and to help shape our own professional futures. There is a need to demonstrate that the nursing profession intends to learn from past experiences and to use its political muscle to good effect in the future under a Labour Government.

The chapters to follow, therefore, will examine six areas of particular interest for all who are concerned to be at the forefront of the developing primary care-led NHS.

CHAPTER 2: REFORMING THE NATIONAL HEALTH SERVICE

This chapter will set the scene for the discussions to follow. It will highlight the period of NHS reform from the early 1980s, the impact of managerial and market changes, culminating latterly in the drift towards a primary care-led NHS, and the subsequent election of a Labour Government in 1997 armed with a new set of health care policies. The developed language, concepts and policy imperatives which have become commonplace to nurses during 18 years of Conservative health administrations will be discussed. In turn, the apparent political reinterpretation of, and emphasis upon the concepts of health, need, patients, collaboration and professionalism, will be set against the backcloth of the reforms and subsequent challenges which have faced nurses during this period. The concluding part will examine new reforms and perspectives offered by the Labour Government for the NHS, and will tentatively propose aspects for further serious consideration by those nurses who are looking for professional development and enrichment in their future nursing lives.

CHAPTER 3: A HEALTHIER NATION

This chapter will reflect back on the promised strategy for health and health care together with an analysis of the reality and intent of Conservative health policy. It will describe the apparent growth and development of a narrow, medicalised, individualistic concept of health and health care. This will be set against the promised notion of a more broadly based, collaborative, environmental vision, as was so glossily promoted in the heavily marketed 'The Health of the Nation' White Paper (Cmd 1986 1992). The positive health focus of that White Paper, presented as ideologically underpinning the NHS reforms, will be shown to have been little more than an illusory, well-packaged idea, limited in scope and intent, and limiting in practice for those many nurses keen to have progressed to a preventive model in health care delivery.

Health and health care will be shown to have been narrowly defined concepts in the internal health care market, more concerned to deal with illnesses than to prevent them. The increasing commercialism of health care activity, and underpinning rationale will be shown to have produced powerful anti-health agendas and inherent dilemmas, with the twin mantras of cost efficiency and proved effectiveness often combining to close down or to ignore any unproved care activity, whatever its imagined potential or apparent relevance and creativity in meeting assessed health need.

The discussion will then turn to look at the agenda of the Labour Government, with its creation of a Minister for Public Health, and an avowed determination not to allow powerful lobbies and vested interests to stand in the way of measures that will ultimately improve health. Such a potentially positive health agenda might open up the possibility for the development of many new interesting professional nurse roles, and even the re-invigoration of some which have visibly wilted because of a clear lack of support in recent years. However, such high expectations for a new health strategy will be set against an examination of the promise to decommercialise the NHS and all that may entail, together with the knowledge that any attempt to deal seriously with the multifaceted causes of ill health, must involve a pan-Whitehall departmental response.

CHAPTER 4: THE CONCEPT OF NEED

The NHS reforms of the 1990s created a context in which the assessment of health need was to play a crucial role in health service planning, providing purchasing bodies with information upon which to build their strategies, to draw up contract specifications for care services, and as a means to evaluate how effectively needs were being met. The discussion in this chapter then will include an examination of the concept of need, and the differences in definition and priority between that of health professionals and lay people. This analysis will be set against the promise for the reforms to create a needs-led service, as opposed to one determined and shaped by professionals.

Initial reference will be made to the National Health Service Management Inquiry of 1983, which offered a damning indictment of the professional self-interest which the Griffiths team believed dominated decision making, and stifled, if not totally ignored, the needs and interests of the uses of health services. The solution put forward by the team, to refocus NHS endeavours in favour of the patients, was the introduction of general management and a more business-like and effective response to consumer need, as apparently provided by successful industries. In addition, the subsequent introduction of the internal health care market following the 1990 National Health Service and Community Care Act established the purchaser–provider split. This provided structures in which an effective commercialised spirit could flourish, and which, it was argued, placed the consumers in a more powerful position to ensure that their needs were met both effectively and to a high standard.

The realities of these intentions will be explored. It will be suggested that there never was any serious intention to define or to respond directly to consumer need, but rather to give the illusion of so doing. The real intent was to contain costs, to limit the health services in breadth of interest and responsibility, to reduce professional power, and to promote a managerial culture with a limited interpretation of what counted as need within the business of the NHS. This limiting agenda will be shown to have impacted on professional development and on the boundaries of practice, and as such to have reduced the ability of nurses to meet the unmet health needs of many groups in the primary health care setting.

Attention will then be drawn towards the present Government's support for a public health vision, an apparently widening focus on health, health service concerns and responsibility. This agenda has the potential within it for professional development, a new expansion of nurse-led activity, with opportunities to develop collective multidisciplinary responses to unmet needs which primary care nurses and others have witnessed in recent years, but have so often been unable to respond to in any meaningful way, if at all, because of a lack of resources and support.

CHAPTER 5: CONSUMER EMPOWERMENT

This chapter will consider the apparent redefinition of the patients/clients of the NHS as consumers in the new commercial-type relationships created by the twin reforms of general managerialism and an internal health care market. The stated intention to strengthen the public's position and the consumer voice will be examined against practice. While some progress may have been achieved, it will become evident that no major effort has been made to develop a stronger user voice.

The claims of the reforms to listen to and respond to consumer preferences, to increase choice and flexibility of care options, will be shown to be little more than a well-packaged ploy to cover up cost containment, retrenchment in services, and a slow dismantling of the previously broadly based responsibility of the NHS. In spite of assertions that the use of charters, increased information and a keenness to listen to consumer voices and needs have increased the quality of services, many professionals and the public alike have noticed a reduction in NHS services – both in quality and quantity. The voices of the public will be shown to have been effectively silenced and ignored.

So, can we look to a better response from the Labour health team? An analysis of their proposals made so far, will be made in order to assess their intention to make the NHS more client centred, and more valuing of the public's views and perceptions of health need. This will be set against the need to challenge the structures created by the reforms, to increase the representation of the public in the decision-making process, and to make appropriate resources available to achieve the changes needed.

CHAPTER 6: NURSING AND PROFESSIONAL DEVELOPMENT

In this chapter we turn to nursing and professional development issues: concerning nurse fears and concerns for nursing as a profession and its likely future. We will reflect upon the heavy challenge to professional nurse credibility during the period of health service reform. Note will be made also of the challenges to professional nurse values, codes of practice and autonomy which became apparent, not least, with information controls being placed on all NHS employees, and on what they might have wished to say openly about the negative impact of the reforms on both patient care and standards. During this period, some would argue that both Government and its political supporters appeared to be orchestrating nurse developments from outside the profession. Trends began to suggest the potential creation of a two-tier body of nurse carers – whether both would be defined as professionals or neither remained to be seen. The new Labour health team of 1997 joined this important debate at a time at which decisions were needed to be made – whether nursing should continue as a distinct profession, or become part of a much wider generic carer structure.

During the immediate post General Election period nurse commentators acknowledged openly the real challenges to their professionalism which nurses had faced on many occasions during the years of the Conservative health reforms. Their code of conduct had often proved difficult to uphold, and it was admitted that too many nurses had not been able to provide the quality and breadth of professional care they would have liked. However, they believed that nurses and their representative bodies were now prepared to start again, and to offer the new Government constructive ideas on how to move the health agenda forward. Members of the nursing profession had much to offer in this respect. They could bring creativity and flexibility to new care agendas. They could give a promise for a serious commitment to working collaboratively with users, managers, other professionals and the politicians, in an effort to work towards a more equitable distribution of health care services than hitherto. In return they would expect to receive the appropriate professional status commensurate with their abilities and knowledge. An analysis of the Government's health policy activity so far will offer some clues as to its response to such a proposition, and to likely developments within the nursing profession in the future.

CHAPTER 7: COLLABORATIVE CARE

The need for a collaborative approach involving professionals, public and politicians alike, is acknowledged by many as a necessary prerequisite for the achievement of good health in society, and for an effective NHS. This chapter will explore the concepts of collaboration and then turn to examine the historical development of it in health care delivery up to the present day. The recent experience of the NHS reforms will be used as the backcloth to a discussion on the many difficulties and barriers to the achievement of effective collaborative ventures – not only within the NHS, but also with other external organisations and with the users of the services.

It will be suggested that those who seek professional development and enrichment of their practice need to look towards a greater understanding of teamworking and collaboration in care. Those nurses who underpin their practice with a philosophy encapsulating collaboration are more likely to achieve professional enhancement than those who continue to work in the old uni-disciplinary team environment, maintaining professional demarcation lines and roles, and offering limited and limiting responses to multi-dimensional health needs.

The Labour Government in its 1997 election manifesto promises for the NHS offered a policy which would help remove some of the structures and organisation barriers to collaborative success, i.e. the fragmented structures and the competitive environment of the internal health care market.

Our fundamental purpose is simple but hugely important: to restore the National Health Service as a public service working co-operatively for patients, not a commercial business driven by competitors.

In turn then, it will be up to all nurses to use the new opportunity offered to make collaboration in care work in the future, and, furthermore, to achieve, or even hold onto, the professional status which is so desired and sought after.

In essence then, as in previous books concerned with nursing and politics, nurses are again being confronted by the often uncomfortable realities of their working lives. They are being challenged to think about these realities in relation to the survival of a nursing profession as they would like it to be – an often difficult task, set as it is against an ever-changing policy backcloth. Inevitably, the vision for today will be replaced by a new perspective on tomorrow. Having acknowledged this, the concluding chapter will discuss some potential future strategies, and encourage, like others before, a collective nurse response.

REFERENCES

Command 1986 1992 The Health of the Nation: a strategy for health in England. HMSO, London
Fatchett A 1994 Politics, policy and nursing. Baillière Tindall, London
Labour Party (Election Manifesto) 1997 Millbank Tower, London
NHSME (National Health Service Management Executive) 1993 A Vision for the Future. Department of Health, London

2

Reforming the National Health Service

The National Health Service (NHS) has experienced a period of great change during the last two decades. This has included the introduction of general management and a more specific managerial approach, together with the creation of an internal health care market. (Griffiths 1983, Cmd 555 1989). These moves have coincided with, and provided the backcloth for, a number of well-promoted and important trends in health care delivery. Significant issues include a strengthened support for collaboration in care and multidisciplinary team working, the achievement of health promotion targets, the empowerment of consumers, the need for researched-based care, the setting of quality standards and audits of clinical effectiveness. Very importantly, these initiatives have developed and grown alongside a proposed change in the power base and focus of health care organisation and delivery from that of the traditional hospital-led service towards a primary health care-led NHS. As Dorrell (Conservative Secretary of Health), described it:

> *The NHS has experienced a process of substantial change over the last few years, beginning with the management reforms launched by 'Working for Patients'. This coincided with significant developments in health policy introduced by the Health of the Nation, the Community Care reforms, the Patient's Charter, the Clinical Effectiveness Initiative and the movement towards a primary care led NHS. The service has come a long way in a short time. (Cmd 3425 1996)*

Towards the end of 1996 primary care was described by Dorrell as fundamental to the NHS. It was people's first point of contact with the service, requiring high quality and strong services to deliver effective and efficient care. He looked to its pivotal role in the developing NHS of the future, providing coordinated care for patients, and multiagency care partnerships, adapting and responding to the specific needs of local communities (Cmd 3512 1996). His proposals, he argued, built on the changes of previous years – 'by giving those closest to the patient, in this case primary care professionals and their teams, a powerful role in improving services' (Cmd 3512 1996).

In turn, the current government has taken up this proposed emphasis in its 1997 White Paper, while setting out its own primary care-led reform programme for the NHS. (Cmd 3807 1997).

SO WHERE ARE WE NOW?

As in the previous period of Conservative health reform, the NHS continues to be an important issue for both political and public debate; providing daily many interesting stories for the whole of the mass media. However, at this early stage of the new Government's life, it is inevitable that debates will continue around the impact of the health policies of its predecessor. The changes made by them will continue to shape the delivery of NHS services for some time to come. Eighteen years of systematic redevelopments in any organisation as large and as complex as the NHS cannot be swept away that easily, even if a totally new approach were to be desired. The reality in practice is likely to be one of incremental change, building upon structures and systems that have been created over time. Some analysis of this process then should help to explain and to check out this Government's commitment to both a primary care-led NHS and to professionals alike. However, before moving on into current debates and responses, much of which is to be raised in later chapters, it is worthwhile reflecting back and reminding ourselves of the background to the reforms in the NHS – changes that have shaped the organisation we find ourselves in today. This chapter will now look at the following:

1. Why we have a national health service.
2. The rise and fall of political consensus and support for a national health service.
3. Demographic and other trends of importance causing concern in the 1970s.
4. Early managerial changes to the NHS.
5. The General Management Inquiry of 1983.
6. Reactions to the Griffiths Report.
7. The NHS review period in 1988.
8. The Conservative Government's strategy for the NHS.
9. 'Working for Patients' (Cmd 555 1989).
10. The internal health-care market: purchasers, providers and contracts.
11. Opposition to the Conservative reforms.
12. Impacts of the reforms.
13. The developing primary health care setting.
14. 'Promoting Better Health' (Cmd 249 1987).
15. 'The GP Contract' (Department of Health 1989).
16. 1992–1997: the Conservative reforms develop.

17. A new approach from a Labour Government.
18. 'The new NHS. Modern, Dependable' (Cmd 3807 1997).

WHY WE HAVE A NATIONAL HEALTH SERVICE

The creation of a national health service after the Second World War represented the rejection of the market-based provision of health care services which had developed over many decades. As with educational provision, housing and employment opportunity, it was acknowledged that individuals 'standing on their own two feet' were not always able to look after themselves or to protect themselves from those uncontrollable external factors which impinged upon their health and well-being, (e.g. economic recession, unemployment, low income, pollution, a dangerous working environment and poor housing). A belief had grown that society should collectively contribute towards the provision of a major institutional social support system. Thus the Welfare State came into being to provide a better balance of opportunity for all citizens, and thus all consumers, to meet their health and social needs. The values underpinning these changes reflected an acknowledgement of, and general responsibility for, each member of society, collectively insuring against the personal, financial and social costs of the unexpected, ill health and other misfortune. Health care and good health were not to be seen as some consumer product to be bought and sold in a market place, or to be dependent upon any one individual's spending power. Also, unlike when buying biscuits, no lay person knew enough about health to choose this or that care. Similarly, unlike returning and complaining about faulty shop goods, it was clearly not easy or indeed in some cases possible to trade in or to question defective care, malpractice or some irreversible life-threatening treatment. The market in health care provision had been a failure for a large part of the population. The new collectivist solution to meeting health care needs for all of the people, and not just for some, was exemplified by the creation of the Welfare State system, including the specific creation of the NHS. It was acknowledged at last that all of the population to a greater or lesser degree needed to be helped to their health care and to good health, and the introduction of the NHS would be the vehicle.

The principles upon which the NHS was established included the following:

1. It was aimed to cover the whole population.
2. It aimed to provide equal access to people in need of health care.
3. It was free at the point of use.
4. It was comprehensive in cover.
5. It was to provide services of a good standard for everyone.
6. It was based on notions of public service.

7. It aimed to be egalitarian in ethos.
8. It aimed to treat individual patients with respect as persons in the collective interest.

The NHS was introduced by the Labour Government in July 1948, in spite of tremendous arguments against it by both Conservative politicians on the opposition benches, and also by many in the medical profession. However, as Michael Foot recalls in his writings about the period, Aneurin Bevan, (Minister of Health in the post-war Labour Government) moved forward in what was described as 'doing the most civilised thing in the world – putting the welfare of the sick in front of other post-war national considerations' (Foot 1973). In similar vein, a nurse called Mary Witting writing in the 'Nursing Times' on July 3rd 1948 said:

> *The great principle has been accepted. Never again need any of us suffer disease through lack of money. Let us be proud that a country still poor after a war has taken this courageous step. It will be responsible for its sick without question, because on the health of each member depends the health of the community. We are part of the service. This is a great time to be alive!*

THE RISE AND FALL OF POLITICAL CONSENSUS AND SUPPORT FOR A NATIONAL HEALTH SERVICE

As we have already noted, the Conservative Party opposed the introduction of the NHS. They assumed a similar approach to other legislation which helped to establish the other important branches of the post-war welfare state. They, however, shifted their position by the time of the 1950 General Election, realising that opposition would reduce their chances of being re-elected. Consequently, the 1950s and 1960s saw a broad political consensus, often called Butskellism, in which the Welfare State and full employment featured as key items in the programmes of all political parties.

The consensus across the political spectrum lasted until the late 1960s when the apparent underperformance of the economy was seen by the political right as resulting from high public spending and direct taxation. Markets, individual freedom and responsibility came back into fashion, leading to the 'Selsdon Man' approach of the Conservatives under Ted Heath's leadership.

While it can be argued that the Heath Government of 1970–74 soon moved back to a consensus approach, the new right wing thinking continued to gain ground. The failure of the Heath Government was blamed by many in the Conservative Party upon its alleged betrayal of right wing policies. With the election of Margaret Thatcher as the Conservative Party leader, a new vigour was given to the encouragement of right wing ideas and policies. As part of what became a new hegemony, the right targeted what they saw as excessive and wasteful public spending. From the late 1970s onwards all public sector bodies, including the NHS, were characterised by the Conservative Government as being under the dead hand of local and central public sector bureaucracies. They were perceived as held back by restrictive practices or powerful professional groups, offering no real consumer choice, demonstrating indifference to quality issues, providing a lack of incentives for innovation and efficiency, and displaying a profound reliance on government funding. In addition, the NHS was seen as a vast and growing consumer of public funds. Indeed it was argued, a variety of problems and challenges directly related to the NHS would, if not addressed, consume more and more of public spending, to the detriment of other important programmes.

DEMOGRAPHIC AND OTHER TRENDS OF IMPORTANCE CAUSING CONCERN IN THE 1970S

In tandem with a hardening of attitudes towards the ever-rising costs of public expenditure on health care was a number of issues which contributed towards these developing concerns. Demographic trends showed increasing numbers of people living to old age and a decline in the ratio of the working population to the non-working population (Central Statistics Office 1993). The subsequent proportional decrease in National Insurance and tax contributions from those of working age would mean that the NHS would increasingly be limited in its ability to meet the expected health care needs of the growing elderly population.

Advances in medical knowledge and technology including new innovations in surgery, drug therapies, screening facilities and diagnostic ability, had in turn created new demands and raised the costs of the NHS in paying for the use of these facilities for its clients. In addition to this, public expectations had risen over time as new possibilities for care have been introduced. People had become better educated and more informed on health and health care matters, and as such had developed as health care consumers, demanding more and more from the NHS: particularly the middle classes (Black 1980). So higher standards of care coupled with increased opportunity for treatment had all combined to push up NHS costs – an outcome not envisaged by Beveridge in the 1940s. He and the other creators of the NHS expected that the cost of the health service would fall as people's needs were met by the new services:

> *With each pair of specs dispensed, each tooth stopped or set of gnashers issued, each ailment cured or chronic disease eliminated, its task and costs*

would be reduced. Beveridge had no conception of medical science as it really is: in a state of dynamic expansion, always devising new health tests for new diseases, new cures and treatments, each more expensive than the last. (Welch 1993)

The new Conservative Government of the late 1970s was clearly aware of all these trends and their long-term impact on public expenditure. While providing reassurance as to the safety of the NHS in their hands, the Government started on the changes which would be necessary for the creation of a new style business-like health service, one which they felt would be better equipped to deal with the health issues and agendas of the 1980s and 1990s.

EARLY MANAGERIAL CHANGES TO THE NHS

The Government looked, it might be argued, to changes which would lead to a 'new contract between public health services and their customers, making a break with the provider-driven, paternalistic welfare approach which had been the dominant modus operandi in health and social care since the Second World War' (Hunter 1993).

Across all welfare institutions, including health, the Government began to push back the boundaries of state provision tightening up, slowing down and reversing the growth in public spending. Some public services were partly or wholly privatised following the introduction of competitive tendering in 1983 (Gaze 1990, Laurent 1990). Increasing use was being made of information technology both to monitor and to distribute health care services, (Luker & Orr 1992). According to Holliday (1992) all aspects of NHS spending were under scrutiny, and efficiency savings were being sought at every opportunity. Of course, none of this is surprising when we reflect on the often expressed scepticism of Margaret Thatcher about state-run services. According to one commentator, she 'never identified with the ideas of the NHS as a public service. Health was a business and as such could learn from the private sector about value for money, service and satisfying "customer" choice' (Dickson 1990). Holliday (1995) noted the following initiatives, which reflected both the Government's intentions to make the NHS more business orientated in approach, and were important precursors to the major management change which was to follow:

◆ Körner Initiatives launched in 1980, designed to improve information systems in the NHS.
◆ Annual efficiency savings decreed by the Secretary of State began in 1981–82.
◆ Annual Review Process launched in 1982 between Secretary of State and Regional Chairs, and Regional Chairs and District Health Authority Chairs, to monitor and to review NHS operations.

◆ Raynor Scrutinies started in 1982 in the NHS. These comprised quick reviews of efficiency in specific areas of the public sector. They made recommendations to secure better value for money.
◆ Central control of manpower from January 1983.
◆ Performance indicators (later to be known as health service indicators) issued from September 1983. These established comparative measures of performance in about 70 areas of clinical work, finance, manpower, support service and estate management.
◆ Forced disposal of surplus NHS property.
◆ Compulsory competitive tendering (CCT) announced in September 1983. CCT forced the NHS to put certain ancillary services out to competitive tender, for example laundry and cleaning work.

The deliberate and concerted introduction of general management into the Health Service which followed these moves was a necessary first part of NHS change, a prerequisite for the reforms to be introduced later, as part of the NHS review of 1988. If the Government wanted to run a market in health care, they needed business people at the helm to make it happen. An inquiry team was set up, therefore, to look at NHS management and to advise the Health Secretary on what action was needed.

THE GENERAL MANAGEMENT INQUIRY OF 1983

The 24-page report of the NHS Management Inquiry Team under the chairmanship of Roy Griffiths (Deputy Managing Director for the food chain J. Sainsburys) was published on 25 October 1983 (Griffiths 1983). Norman Fowler (then Secretary of State for Health), announced in the House of Commons that he accepted the general tenor of the report's findings and recommendations. The inquiry team, consisting of four businessmen, had found at all levels 'a lack of clearly defined general management function, with responsibility too rarely placed on one person' (Fowler 1983). As Griffiths expressed it in his report:

> *If Florence Nightingale were carrying her lamp through the corridors of the NHS today, she would almost certainly be searching for the people in charge.*

The team proposed a series of changes aimed at making the existing organisation work better, which included the identification of general managers regardless of discipline at regional, district and unit levels of the organisation. The general manager would be the final decision maker for issues normally delegated in the past to the consensus management team. This approach, which had existed since the inception of the NHS, was believed by the Inquiry Team to lead to 'lowest common denominator decisions, and long delays in the management process'.

As Griffiths put it in yet another of his colourful analogies:

To the outsider the NHS is so structured as to resemble a mobile: designed to move with any breath of air, but which in fact never changes its position and gives no clear indication of direction.

While denials were made that these proposals represented yet another restructuring of the service, the long-term intentions of the Government for the NHS were as yet unclear. Nevertheless, the Health Secretary's enthusiasm for reform was self-evident in the comments he made to the House of Commons:

The NHS is one of the largest undertakings in Western Europe. The service needs and deserves the very best management we can give it. One of the best contributions we can make to patient care is the improvement in National Health Service Management along the lines recommended by the Griffiths Report.

REACTIONS TO THE GRIFFITHS REPORT

The bodies representing major staff groups in the NHS appeared to accept the team's critique of management, but criticised the introduction of the general management concept. Representative bodies for nurses, the Royal College of Nursing (RCN), the Royal College of Midwives (RCM), the Association of Nursing Administrators (ANA) and the Health Visitors' Association (HVA), saw the report as a snub to the nursing profession (Social Services Committee 1984). Nurses were only mentioned twice in the inquiry report, that is: (1) a facetious remark about Florence Nightingale, and (2) in a passing reference to manpower levels. No real recognition was given to their important role within the NHS, and nowhere in the report was there any recommendation that a senior nurse should have one of the top managerial jobs. The annoyance of the nurse representatives was further compounded by the realisation that Griffiths had flattered and encouraged support from the medical profession by referring to them as 'natural managers at unit level'. So, not only had the nursing profession been badly ignored by Griffiths, but the nurse managers already in post were not even seen as potential contenders for general manager posts. Nurses were outraged at the idea of being managed by a non-health professional who, they felt, would be unable to make decisions on effective patient care, as they believed that 'nurses can only be led and managed by nurses'.

Apart then from specific concerns about the apparent eclipse of nursing by the inquiry team, the Association of Nursing Administrators considered the general manager concept as 'impractical, potentially disruptive and divisive in application' (Social Services Committee 1984). While enthusing about 'rigorous management' and 'crisper decision-making', they defended the well-established consensus management style of the NHS. They implicitly criticised the inquiry team and their commercial approach to management. Unlike a commercial organisation with profit making as a clear objective, they believed the NHS could 'never have a goal any more closely defined than, for example, the best use of health resources or better health for the whole population'. They concluded by saying that: 'decision-making in the NHS needs to be a consensus activity, in which the professional and other specialist interests concerned reach agreement on priorities and policy, and failure in a few areas is not reason to jettison the entire system'. But, in spite of the anti-general management comment made by a wide range of health professionals, including nurses, the new system was introduced.

By the end of the 1980s many NHS employees had had their battles with both the new style NHS management and with the Secretary of State. Nursing staff had gained some representation in the general management hierarchy, but in general had to concede the principle of professional self-government. There was much employee discontent, with nurses among many others taking well-reported industrial action in 1988. A recurrent theme around all the debates was that of the underfunding of the service. The presidents of the medical Royal Colleges gave a warning that acute hospital services were reaching crisis point because of cumulative underfunding, (Hoffenberg, Todd & Pinker 1987). Wards were having to close, and seriously ill babies were among those who were not receiving treatment because of staff and other resource shortages (Butler 1992).

It became increasingly obvious that the Government needed to draw together all of these issues, to provide a political solution which would show leadership and vision, and to prove that the NHS was still safe in their hands. Margaret Thatcher did this, by announcing the review of the NHS during a BBC television programme. According to Turner '. . . within weeks it was evident that this gamble was paying off . . . claims of cumulative underfunding and a complete ministerial muddle were eclipsed by a coherent plan' (Turner 1988).

THE NHS REVIEW PERIOD IN 1988

Clearly much debate ensued about the Government's intentions, and also a variety of opinions was offered as to the correct diagnosis and prescription. Trevor Clay (General Secretary RCN), for example, looked to extra funding and an overhaul of existing NHS structures, as a good way forward. He expressed opposition to those who looked to more radical change, perhaps to systems like those in the USA. He argued that '. . . to have value, alternative structures must provide a better service or, at least, provide the same service at a lower cost . . .' 'Private health insurance', he claimed, 'is expensive to administer, discriminates against the elderly, the poor and the chronically sick and, in the USA has left 40 million people with no medical cover at all' (Clay 1988).

Others disagreed with such arguments and said that increased public funding was not a solution. In spite of the positive effect of the managerial reforms, progress has not been easily made, and thus a new structure was needed. According to Goldsmith (1988), 'the front runner in the debate (was) the internal market where cash follows the patient'. He offered a variety of managed health care ideas which he suggested would provide better working conditions, and a requirement to produce better quality, client-oriented health care, still free at the point of need. He believed that 'every pound put in would then genuinely result in a pound's worth of benefit to the patient rather than fifty penceworth that (appeared) to be provided' at that time.

THE CONSERVATIVE GOVERNMENT'S STRATEGY FOR THE NHS

Only one year after the announcement of the review, the presentation of the Government's strategy for the health service was made to the House of Commons. The contents of the White Paper, 'Working for Patients' (Cmd 555 1989), coupled with those of the Griffiths' Management Inquiry (Griffiths 1983), provided the template for the greatest change in the NHS since its inception in 1948. While the NHS was acknowledged to have provided the seedbed for tremendous advances in medical technology, and a growing menu for treatments to meet the ever-rising demands for health care, this had led to problems. The cost of keeping up with it all was seen as a bit like pouring money down the perpetual black hole. A new way forward had to be adopted.

The general management changes introduced to the NHS in 1984 were seen as a great improvement and very relevant to late twentieth century health care needs. However, new management information systems had revealed clear variations in provision and performance across the country, wide differences in costs, drug prescribing habits, waiting times for operations and in referrals for hospital care by GPs. While there were areas of excellence, the Government stated its intent to raise all hospital and general practice standards to that of the best. They wanted to:

◆ Give patients, wherever they live in the UK, better health care and greater choice of services available.

◆ Give greater satisfaction and rewards to those working in the NHS who successfully respond to local needs and preferences.

Nurses could of course hardly disagree with these objectives, or indeed with many of the other positive statements which characterised the Government's document. It might be worth sifting back through similar health documents of the 1950s, 1960s and 1970s to remind ourselves that all Secretaries of State for Health have stated similar-sounding worthy objectives. What we need to do is to blow away the froth from the top of this particular White Paper and examine the substance. We need to note the problems highlighted, and the solutions on offer, because the means of achieving the changes, and how they are continuing to impact upon nurse practice and client care are central to our concerns today.

'WORKING FOR PATIENTS' (CMD 555 1989)

There was a number of issues raised in the White Paper which the Government perceived as requiring immediate attention. Significantly, the focus of its interest at this stage, as can be seen in the list to follow, appears to be directed at the hospital sector. The emergence of the developing primary care setting as a major focus for care was to become more obvious as the reforms developed.

Problems needing solutions were seen to be:

1. People still sometimes have to wait too long for the treatment and may have little, if any, choice over the time or place at which treatment is given.

2. The service provided on admission to hospital is sometimes too impersonal and inflexible.

It was suggested that all hospitals should provide:

◆ Appointments systems which are reliable.
◆ Quiet and pleasant public waiting areas, with proper facilities for parents with children, and for counselling worried parents and relatives.
◆ Clear information leaflets about the facilities available and what patients need to know when they come into hospital.
◆ Clearer, easier and more sensitive procedures for making suggestions for improvements and, if necessary, complaints.
◆ Once someone is in hospital, clear and sensitive explanations of what is happening – on practical matters, such as where to go and who to see, and on clinical matters, such as the nature of an illness and its proposed treatment.
◆ Rapid notification of the results of diagnostic tests.
◆ A wider range of optional extras and amenities for patients who want to

pay for them, such as single rooms, personal telephones, televisions and a wider choice of meals.

While the last point could be seen by some as describing a two-tier service, the other ideas were clearly less contentious They looked to provide a user-friendly, quality service. Experience suggests that the NHS, organisation and health professionals alike, had failed over time to run and deliver that sort of health service. All the issues raised needed attention whether applied to the hospital or indeed the primary care sector.

Many would feel that in themselves the problems listed so far could have been solved without any drastic reform of the NHS. However the White Paper was not just about dealing with the minutiae of ineffective health care delivery, however important in practice for those on the receiving end. It was in effect proposing major solutions to the problems of funding, controlling and managing a public institution which the Government perceived as being grossly out of control. The White Paper introduced seven key ways of achieving the Government's objectives:

1. The delegation of power and responsibility to local levels – to include greater flexibility in pay and conditions of staff.

2. The creation of self-governing status for hospitals – to be called Trusts.

3. The removal of administrative and financial barriers to enable patients to travel to NHS hospitals of their choice.

4. The reduction of waiting list times both for outpatient and inpatient care by the appointment of more consultants.

5. The ability of large general practices to become budget holders and to compete for patients by offering better services than other practices.

6. The continued improvement of NHS business management effectiveness by the streamlining of management bodies at regional, district and family practitioner levels.

7. The application of rigorous auditing to ensure quality of service and value for money activity throughout the service.

The details of all the major changes were published in a series of working paper (Department of Health 1989), shortly after the White Paper was presented to the House of Commons. Otherwise, the document gave a reasonable flavour of what was to happen in the future. While freeing up the structures and activity of the NHS organisation, the Government also gave explicit support to private sector care, and looked to a new partnership between the public and private sectors. The Government believed that the NHS and independent sector had much to learn from each other, providing both mutual support and services. Any work taken from the NHS, they argued, would not only relieve pressure on it, but offer greater diversity in provision and choice for all. Indeed, the expectation was that there would be further increases in the number of people using private health care services. Unsurprisingly, some believed that these ideas offered clues as to the future direction for NHS development – perhaps to health care privatisation in some form or other. That said, whatever the future intentions at that stage, the success of the Government's proposed changes hinged upon the introduction of a new model for health care provision – the internal health care market.

THE INTERNAL HEALTH CARE MARKET: PURCHASERS, PROVIDERS AND CONTRACTS

This new model for health care delivery replaced the traditional approach in which the NHS was a total provider of services. Previously, the GP, nurse, consultant, hospital or community unit, for example, automatically received payment for services given from the centre. In the new NHS internal health care market however the providers of services were separated from the purchasers, and payment was determined locally through a system of financial contracts. Three types of purchasers therefore came into play:

1. The health authorities.
2. GP fundholders.
3. Private patients.

In addition there were three types of providers:

1. NHS units/hospitals – called Directly Managed Units (DMUs).
2. NHS Trusts – hospitals and community.
3. Private sector units.

Contracting

Within the internal health care market the linking relationship between each of the two sides, purchasers and providers, involved the making of a series of contracts for care. These formal arrangements made at local level thus removed automatic payment from the centre, and provided the means for purchasers to control, to shape and to cost service delivery. Further to this, all providers had to compete with each other for business. This idea was based on the belief that the competitive environment engendered between purchasers and providers would stimulate greater efficiency, raise standards of care and service, and thus place the patient centre stage as the all powerful consumer (Enthoven 1989).

Some of course felt a little uneasy at equating a person seeking health care with a consumer shopping for goods. After all, buying biscuits and clothes are, by definition, different from visiting a doctor or going into hospital for an operation. However, we will return to this particular discussion in a later chapter. The fact is that the introduction of contracting at this stage further extended the cultural shift towards a more business-like approach in the NHS. It was clearly seen as a way of providing some much needed discipline for professionals, who were perceived as profligate users and spenders of public monies. If they wanted their discipline or service to survive, it was up to them as providers to ensure that their contributions to health care were relevant, of high quality, cost effective and efficient, and, above all, consumer friendly. It was up to them to win contracts and to ensure they remained, in effect, in business.

Two major features of the internal health care market included that of the creation of a new kind of provider called the NHS trust, and a new type of purchaser called the GP fundholder.

The hospital trusts – the new providers

One of the important aspects of the creation of the internal health care market was the proposal that as many major acute hospitals (more than 250 beds) as wished to should run their own affairs while remaining part of the NHS. They would be called hospital trusts. While many people will have heard them frequently referred to as opted-out hospitals (i.e. not part of the NHS arrangements), this was repeatedly refuted. As Clarke said in the NHS Review Statement to the House of Commons in January 1989:

Let me make it absolutely clear that they will still be as much within the NHS as they are now. They will be no freer to leave the NHS as they are now. They will be no freer to leave the NHS as any unit has been throughout its forty-year history. (Clarke, 1989a)

The perceived advantages of trust status included:

◆ A stronger sense of local ownership and pride.
◆ An opportunity to build on the enormous fund of goodwill that exists in local communities.
◆ The stimulation of commitment and the harnessing of skills of those who provide the services.
◆ The encouragement of local initiatives.
◆ The development of a greater competitive spirit.

The idea was that hospital trusts would be encouraged to take their own decisions without detailed supervision by district and regional health authorities and the Department of Health. They would be expected to negotiate staff pay rates. They would be able to make contracts to provide care for any purchasers within the NHS, or from the private sector. Subject to the constraints of providing some local essential services, as defined by statute, they would otherwise be able to compete for 'trade' in the national health care market. As finance would now follow patients across authority or regional boundary, the trusts, along with all their new freedoms to manage their own businesses, were bound to redefine and restructure the provision of NHS hospital care. According to the White Paper the hospital trusts would ensure 'a better deal for the public, improving the choice and quality of the services offered and the efficiency with which those services are delivered'.

The budget-holding general practice – the new purchasers

A second proposed major change involved some general practices, if large enough (with lists of initially at least 11 000), becoming budget holders; and thus taking responsibility for purchasing health care services for their patients from either NHS or private sector hospitals. The GPs were seen as having a crucial role in two respects: first, in advising patients and, second, in ensuring that it was the patients who benefited from the reformed health service. By building on the changes in general practice as set out in the earlier White Paper on primary health care (Cmd 249 1987), the new freedoms of activity, it was argued, would allow budget-holding practices to secure better value for money, improve standards of care, offer greater consumer choice, and ensure shorter waiting times for hospital referral and admission for their patients. Practice budgets would encourage shopping around for the best services and employing the right sort of staff to meet the specific needs of the practice. In addition to this, the ability to advertise and develop available practice expertise and services would help attract more patients and thus more money. Savings made because of efficient budgeting could be ploughed back into the practice both to raise standards of service and also to enrich the potential of general practice work for those involved.

All of the activities just described, it was said, would create and sharpen the competitive edge to general practice, and would raise standards as practices would have a clear financial incentive to compete against each other for patients. In addition to this, there was a clear knock-on effect in terms of hospital care from whatever sector. GPs with budgets would only refer to those hospitals which best met the needs of their patients, and which offered them the best value for money. This in turn would create competition between hospitals to gain the contracts. The expected outcome would be a raising of the standards of hospital care offered and also a greater choice of hospitals for patients. The financial incentive to be part of the internal health care market action was made quite clear: 'The practices and hospitals which attract the most customers will receive the most money'. The initial budget-holding practices were to be set up in April 1991 and would be followed by others in succeeding years as the internal health care market developed its activities.

OPPOSITION TO THE CONSERVATIVE REFORMS

Vociferous opposition to the proposed changes came not just from politicians on the Labour and Liberal Democrat benches (Hansard 1989), but from the many and varied nurse interest groups. As one newspaper put it:

> A wall of professional opposition already stands between the Government and the Health Service. It begins to look more impregnable day by day. Hospital consultants, nurses and GPs are all opposed to the Government's proposed restructuring of the NHS. So are the institutions: not just their unions – the BMA, NUPE and COHSE – but nine Royal Medical Colleges and the Royal College of Nursing as well. (Editorial 1989)

According to Clay (1989a), the proposed reforms were not seen as tackling a new health agenda, but preoccupied with issues of management and financial accountability. It was acknowledged by many that the market philosophy would increasingly change the character of the NHS in ways which were unpredictable at that stage. Rowden (1989) and many other nurse commentators also drew attention to the possibility of cost-cutting exercises, the avoidance of caring for vulnerable or chronically ill people to avoid high long-term expenditure, the increasing workload of nurses outside hospital coping with enlarging popular practices, 'quicker and sicker' discharges from hospital following a speedier throughput of clients after surgery, and even the possibility of nurses being employed as 'mini-doctors' to reduce medical costs. The fears and concerns, therefore, were many at this stage.

The further details of the major changes which were set out in the eight Working Papers (Department of Health 1989), published after the White Paper, were greeted with yet more opposition. In a strongly worded statement following their publication, Clay, RCN General Secretary, said:

> These papers leave too many questions unanswered. It appears that the brakes are off. A much wider range of hospitals and even community services will be able to opt for trust status. (Clay 1989b)

The debate was clearly developing fast and furiously both for and against the proposals. No one working in the NHS at that time will have failed to notice it. Calls for nurses to stop the progress of the reforms were made because, as argued by Storey, RCN President, in April 1989: 'The package as a whole jarred against fundamental NHS principles of equity, comprehensiveness and balance' (Storey 1989). However, the Health Secretary at the very same Conference at which Storey spoke said: 'No one should have any doubt that the reforms of the National Health Service are going to happen' (Clarke 1989b).

By this stage, many who opposed the reforms, both public and health professional alike, were engaging themselves in campaigns using all possible media outlets in their workplaces, and via local and national protest groups. Nurse and doctor representative organisations played their part highlighting concerns about reductions in standards of care, a need for more resources and fears for the future of the NHS. Opposition politicians took their arguments to the floor of the House of Commons and challenged the Health Secretary at every available opportunity. Government supporters in turn described opposition tactics as 'misinformation and lying attacks, a mindless barrage of propaganda and an outrageous campaign of frightening little old ladies' (Rawnsley 1989). The Health Secretary, in response, reiterated time after time promises of success for the reforms. He argued that:

Doctors will not run out of money, preventing them from prescribing treatments; GPs will not be under pressure to devote less time to patients; essential local hospital services will be safeguarded, quality of care, not cost will be the decisive factor in doctors' decision-making; and the Government's commitment to the health service is absolute and will remain so. (Clarke 1989c)

By July 1989 Kenneth Clarke had written to all levels of management to request that they ensure their staff were kept fully informed of the true nature of the changes so as to avoid staff being upset by persistent rumours and misinformation promulgated by anti-Government commentators. One doctor had resigned from his long-term membership of the BMA, arguing that 'frightening the patient is not part of the Hippocratic oath'. He felt the BMA campaign had created specious fears about whether or not people, particularly the elderly, would have to travel hundreds of miles to get a hospital bed, or whether their doctors would be able to offer to prescribe drugs they needed (Lockley 1989).

The discussions and arguments were further fired by the publication of 'Caring for People' (Cmd 849 1989). Community care plans were also going to follow the market approach to purchasing and providing care. Not surprisingly, accusations again flowed as to the applicability of this model to the provision of community care. In addition to this, the effective split being created between health and social care provision was seen as fraught with untold problems.

1990: a new year and new arguments

Headlines of concern followed one after another as the debate hotted up around the introduction of the NHS internal health care market with its purchasers and providers. The budget-holding notion for GPs was seen as flawed according to a group of American health experts. They argued that 'The Government's proposals require changes if they are to work as expected and are not to jeopardise standards of patient care'. (Brindle 1990a). In March, further fuel was added to the flames when it was announced that 'outsiders had been brought in to drive through the Government's controversial health reforms' (Brindle 1990b). However, one appointee to the Chair of South Manchester District Health Authority with clear management experience in brewing said, 'the NHS is not a business, but that does not mean it cannot benefit from business methods. More services and improved quality would result from increasing efficiency and encouraging customer awareness.'

The NHS and Community Care Act 1990

In June 1990 the NHS and Community Care Act became law. The acrimonious debates continued, particularly when it was announced in July that the Community Care changes would be phased in over 3 years to start formally in April 1993. On the other hand, the internal health care market was to start the following year in April 1991, without pilot or trials. Some thought that it was a very unscientific way of doing things and certainly contrary to normal good practice in the NHS.

The preparations for the new internal market arrangements developed quickly during the following months. Interestingly, the new Health Secretary, William Waldegrave, expressed some concern at the business jargon which appeared to be over-running the NHS. One commentator queried the ability of patients of the future being able 'to tell the difference between a hospital and a supermarket. Whilst there were no waiting lists at Asda's or Sainsbury's, the language used by those in charge of the NHS was becoming very similar to that used in shops' (Editorial 1990). Indeed, another commented that 'the White Paper contained some choice examples of language which reduced the whole process of health care to movements of money and the generation of paperwork' (Downe 1990).

By March 1991 the NHS was poised for lift-off. But, behind the outward show from Government of a smooth and purposeful transition, lay apparently a great deal of chaos, confusion and uncertainty. The earlier suggested promise of a truly sharp competitive edge to the new health care purchaser–provider relationships had slowly been calmed down, both in language used by Government, and also in what was to be allowed to happen in the first year. According to Butler (1992) there was to be 'smooth continuity with the past rather than sharp divergence from it'. It was clearly felt imperative that there should be as few obvious embarrassments or problems for the Government during year one of the introduction of the changes. The market approach could not be allowed to let rip – yet. By March 1991 the NHS was ready for a 'steady' lift-off. It had the structures and the management with business skills – but did it have the support of the staff?

Feelings before lift-off – 1 April 1991

According to a survey of nursing staff, many were voicing concern on the eve of the reforms (Snell & Gaze 1991):

◆ 60% of nurses questioned believed reforms would not improve patient care.
◆ Over half questioned were against the reforms.
◆ A large proportion felt that nursing would suffer at the ward/unit and district level after 1 April 1991.
◆ Nurses in Wales feared the impact of purchaser–provider contracts had been underestimated.
◆ Staff in Cardiff claimed a night dialysis service was under threat because it was expensive and uncompetitive in the new purchaser–provider world.
◆ Staff in Northwest Surrey Health Authority working in the mental handicap unit were confused and concerned about the prospect of trust status.
◆ In Trent, COHSE members confirmed their opposition to reforms.
◆ Nurses in Scotland expressed the hope that they would be able to learn from mistakes in England and Wales as they did not implement their changes until April 1992.

Clearly, while these points only represent some of the comments made, they give a feel of the concern expressed by many nurses. On 31 March the Health Secretary tried to reassure both health professional and public alike.

There is going to be a great deal of talk. The turmoil is going to make a lot of people uncomfortable. But I'm confident that it will come out right in the end. (Waldegrave 1991)

IMPACTS OF THE REFORMS

By May 1991 it was reported that the Government's new health market in the NHS was running into serious difficulties, and patients were paying the price. Huge variations in the cost of operations became apparent, and an embryonic two-tier system emerged in general practice with the budget-holders getting better deals for their patients at the expense of non-budget-holders. Patient choice was also being restricted, because health authorities did not necessarily have contracts with specific hospitals chosen, (Ferriman 1991).

One district health authority in Kent would not pay for a woman to have a sterilisation operation in Guy's Hospital and another woman in Lothian was refused in vitro fertilisation (Harman 1991). Family doctors in Coventry were told that even if patients had spent years on waiting lists, they could not be referred outside contracted hospitals. The contracting process was also rais-ing ethical questions. The chairman of a senior consultants' body said that hospital consultants who agreed to give preference to patients whose GPs were budget-holders could be referred to the General Medical Council for unethical conduct (Mihill 1991). The Health Secretary acknowledged that the changes were indeed bringing about inequalities, but that all the unfairness thrown up by the changes should be borne because of the eventual benefits (Travis 1991).

Support for the Government

A leading Conservative health advisor (Baroness Cumberlege) spoke out against all the opposition to change, accusing those who did so of destroying the NHS: 'My concern is that the NHS is in danger of following the path of British Leyland: every union is scoring points by denigrating the service; mar-ket share is declining; confidence is ebbing, we are following that awful down-hill path to self-destruction that has been trodden before.' (Brindle 1991a). Some might perceive that this was a novel way of deflecting blame away from some of the negative reports of the Government's reforms – the unhappy out-comes of which stayed firmly on the agenda. While NHS changes were accused of 'hampering health care' (Brindle 1991b), the Government's own research published shortly after came up with very different conclusions.

1992 – good news, bad news

At the beginning of the year the DoH circulated reports showing that patients believed trusts were a good thing, and also that the reforms in the first 6 months were found to be working successfully (NHS Management Executive 1991, Hamblin 1992). However, for many the headline 'Fury of Tory Surgeon Who Says Reforms Killed Patients' (Ferriman 1992) seemed in sharp contrast to the Government's own report and assessment.

The gradual build up to the April General Election started well before the announcement of it by the Prime Minister. The impact of the NHS changes had provided the meat of political debate for all the major parties for months.

The General Election – April 1992

The campaign itself highlighted arguments both for and against the NHS reforms. Many will remember the furore over the 'Jennifer's ear' story (Hencke 1992). While it has been suggested that it rebounded on the Labour Party, nonetheless it highlighted some of the problems of the internal health care market, including the inequities of care provision already noted, and the alleged immorality of a two-tier health care system which allowed those with money to jump the queue, while others were forced to wait. The outcome of the General Election, however, ensured that all was 'full steam ahead' in the

NHS. The Conservative Government had been given another 5 years to develop their internal health care market.

THE DEVELOPING PRIMARY HEALTH CARE SETTING

Simultaneously, and centrally to these major changes in the NHS, appeared to be the developing power of the primary health care setting. While at the inception of the NHS and certainly during the 1950s and 1960s the role and status of the hospital sector was paramount, during the 1970s and 1980s the future powerful role of primary health care was slowly becoming more evident. This trend was probably as a result of the already mentioned desire of the Conservative Government both to constrain and to cut public expenditure. The ever-rising costs of acute hospital-based care were perceived to be out of control, and would, if not reined in, swallow up resources needed for other important areas. There was a belief that the 'gate-keeper' role of general practice, could, if it were tightened up and developed along managerial lines, play an important part in holding down the ever-rising costs of health care delivery. General practitioners and their teams were to play a key role in deciding who should get what, where and how within the reforming health service. Some of the roots of such developments can be traced back to the publication of the Government's White Paper, 'Promoting Better Health' in 1987. (Cmd 249 1987)

'PROMOTING BETTER HEALTH' (CMD 249 1987)

The document set out the Government's intent to improve primary health care delivery based on the development of general practice as the focus for care. The onus was placed on the then family practitioner committees (now health authorities) to ensure that primary health care delivery within general practice teams would develop in a number of important ways. Efforts were to be made to ensure the following:

◆ To make services responsive to needs.
◆ To ensure the widest range of choice for care.
◆ To monitor and improve the quality of care.
◆ To set clear priorities for care.
◆ To ensure value for money.
◆ To give special attention to health promotion and illness prevention.

It was believed that primary health care teams (PHCTs) had the ability and the potential to meet these responsibilities within realistic financial and professional frameworks. In turn this was likely to generate better quality services, producing efficient and effective care and treatment for individuals, families and communities alike.

THE NEW GP CONTRACT 1989

Following the White Paper (1987) a new contract of employment for GPs was negotiated during 1988–1989. First, it aimed to focus GP activity on improving patient choice and on raising standards of care offered. It ratified the strengthening NHS focus on health promotion and illness prevention and included the requirement for:

◆ Screening targets.
◆ Health promotion clinics.
◆ Regular health check-ups – particularly for vulnerable people.

Second, the contract provided a degree of control by the centre on general practice. It included the introduction of indicative prescribing and the monitoring of such. Medical audit by a peer review system was started, with the requirement for much closer monitoring of all GP activity. Practices had to in effect 'set out their stalls' by providing information on the services they had to offer, as well as their team's qualifications and ability to provide them. Standards for good practice also had to be defined and the means to determine the degree of achievement reached to be clearly set out. Specific hours of working, a 24-hour responsibility for patients and a requirement to live at a reasonable distance from practices were also put into the contract.

The process of contract negotiation and agreement between Kenneth Clarke and the BMA during 1988/89 was to say the least a fraught experience. The financial incentives provided within it, to encourage GPs to develop their practice and services in line with the Government's approach, hit many raw nerves. One speaker at a BMA Conference summed up her colleagues' derision for Mr Clarke and for the Government's reforming plans:

> *Oh dear Mr Clarke*
> *You're not quite so smart*
> *As Maggie would have us believe*
> *Forget your incentives*
> *You're not that inventive*
> *We GPs are not that naive.*

In spite of the many and varied protests the new contract was published in the summer of 1989, and it was implemented from 1 April 1990. As noted by many commentators the contract resulted in significant increases in GP's incomes. In turn the new requirements, not least around health promotion, saw the development of many new interesting employment opportunities for nurses within general practice: a trend which continues to this day.

With the subsequent impact of the reforms of the 1990s, and specifically the developments in GP fundholding, it was to become very clear that general practice was a central rather than peripheral platform for health care delivery in the NHS of the future.

1992 TO 1997 – THE CONSERVATIVE REFORMS DEVELOP

The period from April 1992 to 1996 saw the further development and consolidation of many of the internal market mechanisms already noted. The apparent 'completion' of these was on 1 April 1996. According to Dorrell (Dorrell 1996), it marked 'the end of the process of institutional upheaval launched in the 1990s, which was designed to ensure the health service was more efficiently and more responsibly run'. The issue now paramount was how to use the new structures to deliver the kind of health service people wanted, to move away from arguments about managerialism, and to address important questions about the provision of quality services and the changed shape of health care delivery.

In a sense he was determined to look forward, not least because he believed the changes, while highly controversial at the time, had been accepted as a permanent part of the NHS landscape. Indeed, Dorrell was pleased to note that a report by the Association of Community Health Councils, an unusual ally, accepted that 'the changes had partially succeeded in their aim of combating the sense of financial crisis in the NHS and the political pressure which this used to create'. Unsurprisingly, many health professionals, including nurses, disagreed with this. For them, far from becoming a more peaceful process, the whole period since 1992 had witnessed intense political argument, the focus of which was often that of the difficulties created by financial pressures, for example rationing and rationalisation of health care services, closures of hospitals and wards, winter bed crises, a lack of intensive care beds and professional nurse redundancies. Brindle (Dorrell 1996) refers to the period as one of 'revolution' in light of all that has taken place, and the changes made – some for the better, some for the worse. Appleby (1996) interestingly observed that 'although in some narrow legislative sense the reforms might be over, in a wider (and more real) sense change was ongoing'. He noted that the reforms had a long way to go: managerially in how the jobs of purchasing, providing, regulating, etc. are performed, and culturally in the way that the new economic environment was perceived and understood by the key actors in the NHS. In a sense then, throughout 1996, and into 1997 for that matter, many were still having to come to terms with very profound changes in their working lives as NHS professionals. Indeed, any cursory re-read of the 'Working for Patients' White Paper of 1989, and its almost skeletal framework for reform, only serves to bring home to the reader the enormous conceptual leaps that have been taken by those within the organisation since 1992.

What has happened since 1992?

After the re-election of a Conservative Government in 1992, the NHS reforms have developed apace.

◆ The concept of trust status was applied not just to the hospital setting, but to community units and to the ambulance services alike.

◆ The increasingly commercialised focus for health service delivery saw the development of skills in pricing, purchasing, contracting, quality standard setting and auditing of all care interventions.

◆ The importance of proving the value of all care activity resulted in a much greater emphasis on the need to use research findings to underpin all work, and to the development of research initiatives to ensure that practice is evidence based.

◆ There has been a programme of rationalisation throughout the whole of the hospital sector, with closures and mergers increasingly evident across the UK, including London.

◆ The 14 statutory regional health authorities (RHAs) have been abolished and replaced by eight regional offices of the National Health Service Management Executive (NHSME).

◆ District health authorities (DHAs) have merged with their local family health services authorities (FHSAs), to create stronger local purchasers bodies, and are now referred to as health authorities (HAs)

◆ The primary health care-led NHS focus as suggested earlier has become even stronger over time. The early GP budget-holding processes have developed into a number of influential models, including multifund purchasing, total fundholding and care-holding, (Dinsdale 1998).

In addition, the competitive relationship between practices engendered by the reforms has influenced a massive growth in general practice services now available to their clients. Some now carry out a range of minor operations, others employ hospital consultants to provide a service in the practice building which would previously only have been available in an outpatient department clinic. Added to this, the use of new information systems, desktop communication, processing, publishing, prescribing and pathology systems have all combined to build up practice information, and to expedite and to facilitate general practice care and services.

In very general terms the gradual empowerment of general practice and the primary health care team (PHCT) as a focus for care, has influenced the ways in which the hospital sector has worked and developed during the reforms. The placing or non-placing of contracts has been a powerful tool, not least in relation to the strongest and weakest of hospitals all competing for business in the internal market. The hospital sector is general, and not least the powerful consultant-led teams, (both medical and surgical) have had to woo the interests of the purchasers, metaphorically 'outside of their hospital walls'. New and interesting vertical outreach team working has developed, ideally to provide continuity of care for patients, and to develop liaison effectiveness from hospital to community and vice versa. Another pressing reality of course, has been the need to secure good relationships with the purchaser bodies (and not least the GPs) and to gain a competitive edge and market lead over other nearby provider bodies with similar care interests and packages on offer.

As purchasers, GP fundholders have been able to select from a broad menu of care services to meet the varied and wide health needs of their practice clientele: from prescribing a course of sessions at a sports centre, for example, to surgical or medical or other interventions in the most appropriate and cost-effective venue. In a sense, the traditional gate-keeper role of general practice has been enhanced at the expense of the powerful secondary sector and hospital-led consultant services. In turn the requirement for general practice teams to apply a positive health focused agenda, for example 'Promoting Better Health' (1987), 'The Health of the Nation' (1992), 'The GP Contract' (1990), has led to a stronger focus on health, health promotion, illness prevention and health education initiatives, and the provision of alternative therapies, rather than to immediate reliance on drugs and referral to the hospital sector. Holliday (1995) described this trend as indicating that:

> *The medical definition of disease, centred on glamour services provided by hospital consultants has been coming under scrutiny and challenge as a transfer of emphasis from secondary to primary care takes place.*

Therefore by 1996 the direction of the reforms was firmly pointing to general practice as the major focus for care. The primary care-led NHS as described by Dorrell at the beginning of the chapter was clearly now on line, and the continuing developments he sought after 1 April of that year related directly to general practice and the primary health care teams. As can be imagined, the particular pre-election support for a primary care-led NHS, and its professional carers, was well received by many. For those in primary health care employment, the future looked potentially both optimistic and very interesting. As the new year progressed, and the General Election drew nearer, the political debates around the NHS developed, with each political party setting out its differing manifesto promises (Health Services Journal 1997). The assumption made by most health commentators, however, was that even if there were a politically different team at the Department of Health after the

General Election, many of the health reforms were unlikely to be fundamentally revised, although the emphasis they took was likely to change.

A new Conservative Government, it was said, would herald a continuation of encouragement for competition between health providers, and an increasing development of a mixed economy of provision. On the other hand, if Labour were to win, there was an expectation of increased move to more centralised planning, and attempts to create a more equitable delivery of health care than hitherto. All commentators however appeared to agree on one point – whichever Government was returned, there would be continued policy adjustments and change.

On 2 May 1997, the Conservatives lost the General Election and were replaced by a Labour Government. As such the plans and ideas of the previous Government were no longer in the ascendancy. Unfortunately (but perhaps inevitably), the Conservative's NHS reforms of over nearly two decades had left for many professionals a legacy of suspicion and doubt about the future of the NHS, and their role within it. A great number had become increasingly cynical, and their morale had plummeted as the reforms had developed (Traynor 1995). Too often they had been made to feel marginalised as managerial developments and processes took hold of the organisation. Meads (1996) referred to professionals' views as having been too often 'bypassed or even, on occasion, alienated by official explanations of reforms that have concentrated on the mechanisms of change, rather than their underlying values or intended outcomes'. The new government would clearly need to convince many professionals as to the sincerity of their promise to listen more closely to their views.

A NEW APPROACH FROM A LABOUR GOVERNMENT

After 18 years in opposition the newly elected Labour Government of 1997 and its health team clearly faced a difficult agenda. They had the demanding task of both reviewing and changing a very well-established political approach and ideology underpinning the management and delivery of health care in the UK. As Dickson described it:

> *The new Secretary of State for Health, Frank Dobson, has been handed one of the most difficult portfolios in Whitehall. (Dickson 1997)*

Within 12 days of the General Election result a broad vision was given in the Queen's speech of proposed initial changes to be implemented in the NHS under a Labour Government. These included:

◆ An end to the internal health care market.

◆ The replacement of GP fundholding with GP commissioning.
◆ A reduction in the number of bureaucrats.
◆ Shorter waiting lists for treatment.
◆ A moratorium and a new review of London hospital closures.
◆ A national minimum wage for NHS employees.
◆ Investigation into national pay frameworks.
◆ Overhaul of 'The Health of the Nation' document.
◆ Creation of a ban on tobacco advertising.
◆ Overhaul of 'The Patient's Charter'.
◆ Royal Commission on continuing care arrangements.
◆ Review of the private finance initiatives.

At this very early stage, the Government set out an initial agenda of change for the NHS, the details of which would appear as time moved on, and against which the public and professional alike would be able to judge the sincerity of the promises made so soon after the General Election. It was to be five months before the promised White Paper on the future of the NHS was published.

'THE NEW NHS MODERN, DEPENDABLE' (CMD 3807 1997)

The opening statement of the December White Paper very much set the scene for the detail to follow:

> *The government is committed to giving the people of the country the best system of health care in the world. At its best the National Health Service is the envy of the world. But often it takes too long for patients to get treated. Quality is variable. And NHS staff feel too much of their time and effort is diverted from treating patients into pushing paper. This White Paper explains how the Government working with those one million staff, will build a modern and dependable health service fit for the twenty-first century. A national health service which offers people prompt, high quality treatment and care when and where they need it. An NHS that does not just treat people when they are ill, but works with others to improve health and to reduce inequalities. (Cmd 3807 1997)*

The general approach was very much concerned to conserve what had worked and to discard the rest. It was acknowledged at the outset that not everything about the previous system was bad. The separation between the planning and providing of care, for example, was to be maintained, but the competitive nature of the internal health care market was to go. While it had been seen as a way to improve care delivery for all, it was believed to have created more problems than it had solved. The 1997 White Paper lists a number of such issues:

◆ Fragmentation of services.
◆ Unfairness.
◆ Distortions.
◆ Inefficiencies.
◆ Heavy bureaucracy.
◆ Instability.
◆ Secrecy.

In general, it was argued that the competitive focus of the internal health care market mechanisms and processes, had resulted in a side-tracking of resources from health care to administration. The NHS had therefore been prevented from properly focusing on the needs of the patients. As the White Paper pointed out:

> *The internal market was a misconceived attempt to tackle the pressures facing the NHS. It has been an obstacle to the necessary modernisation of the health service. It created more problems than it solved. This is why the Government is abolishing it.*

A new approach therefore was to be introduced over a period of 10 years, one which aimed to avoid the organisational upheavals and failures of previous years:

> *There will be no return to the old centralised command and control systems of the 1970s. That stifled innovation and put the needs of institutions ahead of the needs of patients. Nor will there be a continuation of the divisive internal market system of the 1990s. That approach which was intended to make the NHS more efficient, ended up fragmenting decision-making and distorting incentives to such an extent that unfairness and bureaucracy became its defining features.*

The NHS of the future was thus to be run in a 'third way', a system which was based on 'partnership and driven by performance'. It was described as 'a new model for a new century'.

Six important principles were to underlie all the changes:

◆ To review the NHS as a genuinely *national* service, with patients receiving access to consistently high quality, prompt and accessible services right across the country.

◆ To make the delivery of health care against these new standards a matter of *local* responsibility. Local doctors and nurses who are in the best position to know what patients need will be in the driving seat in shaping services.

◆ To get the NHS to work in *partnership*. By breaking down organisational barriers and forging stronger links with local authorities, the needs of the patient will be put at the centre of the care process.

◆ To drive *efficiency* through a more rigorous approach to performance and by cutting bureaucracy, so that every pound in the NHS is spent to maximise the care for patients.

◆ To shift the focus onto quality of care so that *excellence* is guaranteed to all patients and quality becomes the driving force for decision making at every level of the service.

◆ To rebuild *public confidence* in the NHS as a public service, accountable to patients, open to the public and shaped by their views.

While then providing a number of key themes to underpin all developments in the future, it proposed two broad elements of activity:

1. The separation between the planning of hospital care and its provision will be retained. 'By empowering local doctors and nurses and Health Authorities to plan services, this will ensure that the local NHS is built around the needs of patients. While hospitals and other agencies providing services will have a hand in shaping these plans, their primary duty will be to meet patients' requirements for high quality and easily accessible services.'

2. The increasingly important role of primary care will be developed. As the White Paper explained:

> *Most of the contact that patients have with the NHS is through a primary care professional such as a community nurse or family doctor. They are best placed to understand their patients' needs as a whole and to identify ways of making local services more responsive. Family doctors who have been involved in commissioning services (either as fundholders, or through multi-funds, locality commissioning or the total purchasing model) have welcomed the chance to influence the use of resources to improve patient care. The Government wishes to build on these approaches, ensuring that all patients, rather than just some, are able to benefit.*

The responsibility for the operational management of these approaches is to be decentralised to allow NHS trusts help shape the locally agreed framework which will determine how NHS services develop. In the future, it is argued, the approach will be one of interdependence rather than independence and fragmentation of care responses. The 10-year modernisation programme thus offers a number of important proposals to improve efficiency, to develop new models for primary care delivery, to enhance and sharpen the work of trusts, to find new ways of providing effective collaborative multidisciplinary health care initiatives at local levels, and to manage better the costs of the services provided. The Government acknowledged it was a tough and challenging programme:

On some fronts there will be early progress. Others may be for the long-haul. Some may take time to show visible improvement. But the end result will be an NHS that responds to a changed and changing world.

According to Margaret Jay (Health Minister with responsibility for nursing): 'The White Paper, "The New NHS" sets out the government's commitment to giving the people of this country a modern and dependable health service. To achieve this, partnership with the million people who work in the health service is essential. Crucially, it means partnership with nurses.' (Jay 1997).

CONCLUSION

At this early stage of the Government's life, and indeed that of a new NHS reform programme, there is inevitably a large number of questions left unanswered:

◆ Will the new approach be better than the internal health care market?
◆ Will the service be truly health focused and needs led?
◆ Will multidisciplinary collaborative care ventures really work?
◆ Will the users of the NHS become the central focus for care?
◆ Will their voices be better heard?

These questions will undoubtedly become part of the political debate around the success of the new health agenda. They are also equally relevant to nurses, not least in determining whether the NHS under this new Government will provide the context in which the shared and communal values of professional nursing can be effectively implemented and developed. The discussions in the following chapters will hopefully go some way towards clarifying nursing's present position, and to planning a hopefully successful professional future in NHS 2000.

REFERENCES

Appleby J 1996 The Reforms. Health Service Journal 13 June
Black D 1980 Inequalities in health. Report of a research working group. HMSO, London
Brindle D 1990a Budget plan for GP's 'flawed'. The Guardian, 26 January
Brindle D 1990b Outsiders picked to oversee health service changes. The Guardian 12 March
Brindle D 1991a Health chief warns of NHS path to ruin. The Guardian 7 June
Brindle D 1991b NHS changes 'hampering health care'. The Guardian 7 November
Butler J 1992 Patients, policies and politics. Open University Press, Milton Keynes
Central Statistical Office 1993 Social Trends 23. HMSO, London
Clarke K 1989a Statement NHS review. Hansard, 146(39): 31 January
Clarke K 1989b In: Brindle D. Reforms will go forward, Clarke warns nurses. The Guardian 4 April
Clarke K 1989c In: Brindle D. Clarke tells GPs of leaflet errors. The Guardian 20 April

Clay T 1988 What treatment does the NHS need? Nursing Times 84(16): 34

Clay T 1989a Clay on the review. Nursing Times 85(6): 21

Clay Trevor 1989b In: News: Working Papers 'a backward step' say nursing unions. Nursing Times 85(9): 6

Command 249 1987 Promoting Better Health. Department of Health, London

Command 555 1989 Working for patients. Department of Health, London

Command 849 1989 Caring for People. Department of Health, London

Command 3425 1996 The National Health Service: a service with ambitions. Department of Health, London, November

Command 3512 1996 Primary care: delivering the future. Department of Health, London, December

Command 3807 1997 The New NHS. Modern, dependable. Department of Health, London

Department of Health 1989 General practice in the NHS: The 1990 contract. HMSO, London

Department of Health 1989 National Health Service review working papers. (Package of 8 booklets). HMSO, London

Dickson N 1990 The Thatcher legacy. Nursing Times 86(48): 22

Dickson N 1997 Dobson's choice. Nursing Times 93(21): 22

Dinsdale P 1998 Pilot lights new way forward. The Guardian. 4 February, 7

Dorrell S 1996 In: Brindle D. After the revolution, a time for peace. The Guardian 3 April

Downe Soo 1990 Ward power. Nursing Times 86(16): 24

Editorial 1989 The support is not there. The Guardian 28 March

Editorial 1990 Comment. Nursing Times 86(51): 3

Enthoven A 1989 In: Robinson R. New health care market. British Medical Journal 298: 437–439

Ferriman A 1991 Patients pay price of the market. Sunday Observer 5 May

Ferriman A 1992 Fury of Tory surgeon who says reforms killed patients. Sunday Observer 9 February

Foot M 1973 Aneurin Bevan, vol 2. Davis Poynter, London

Fowler N 1983 Hansard (1286): 168

Gaze H 1990 Sweeping change? Nursing Times 86(24): 27–28

Goldsmith M 1988 The case for a radical overhaul. Nursing Times 84(16): 35

Griffiths R 1983 The NHS management inquiry report. Letter to Norman Fowler. Department of Health, London

Hamblin M 1992 Attitudes among patients leaving Trust hospitals. Department of Health, London

Hansard 1989 Statement on NHS review. Hansard 146(39): 165–189

Harman H 1991 Reform that will end in tiers. The Guardian 21 May

Health Services Journal 1997 It's party time. 10 April, pp 12, 13

Hencke D 1992 Couple divided on broadcast. The Guardian 26 March

Hoffenberg R, Todd I P, Pinker G 1987 Crisis in the National Health Service. British Medical Journal 295: 1505

Holliday I 1995 The NHS transformed, 2nd edn. Baseline Books, Manchester

Hunter D 1993 To market! To market! A new dawn for community care. Health and Social Care in the Community 1(1): 3–10

Jay M 1997 The White Paper recognises that nurses have a critical contribution to make. Nursing Times 93(51): 3

Laurent C 1990 Taken to the cleaners? Nursing Times 86(19): 20

Lockley J 1989 Advice from the BMA that patients should ignore. The Guardian 18 September

Luker K, Orr J (eds) 1992 Health visiting. Towards community health nursing. Blackwell Scientific Publications, Oxford

Meads G (ed) 1996 A primary care-led NHS. Churchill Livingstone, Edinburgh

Mihill C 1991 NHS contract deal raises ethics threat. The Guardian 4 May

NHS Management Executive 1991 NHS reforms. The first six months. HMSO, London

Rawnsley A 1989 Overweight Health Minister ignores doctors' orders. The Guardian 26 April

Rowden R 1989 What's in it for us? Nursing Times 85(8): 45

Snell J, Gaze H 1991 Staff across the UK voice concern on the eve of health service reforms. Nursing Times 87(13): 8

Social Services Committee 1984 Griffiths NHS management inquiry report, 1983–84. HC 209. HSMO, London

Storey M 1989 In: Brindle D. Reforms will go forward, Clarke warns nurses. The Guardian 4 April

Traynor M 1995 Job satisfaction and morale of nurses in NHS Trusts. Nursing Times 91(26): 42–44

Travis A 1991 Health Secretary admits new inequalities. The Guardian 27 May

Turner T 1988 The last nail. Nursing Times 84(16): 28–30

Waldegrave W 1991 In: Koenig P, Kingman S, Sage A. The NHS and you. The Independent on Sunday 31 March

Welch C 1993 Now the bourgeoisie bang their spoons. The Independent 31 May

3

A healthier nation

The health problems facing the community are too urgent and too large in scale to allow complacency. Every year in Europe millions die prematurely or suffer ill health from serious conditions that could have been prevented. At the same time health systems throughout the Community are coming under increasing strain as a result of the mounting demands being made upon them and the difficult financial situation that member states are facing. The pressures of having to cope with rapidly changing medical technology, with an ageing population with ever-growing needs for health care and social support, and with people's constantly rising expectations about health services are therefore forcing member states to take sweeping measures to reform their health systems and to control costs. (Pádraig Flynn 1997; Member of the European Commission, Responsibility for Employment and Social Affairs)

Over the past decade and a half successive UK Conservative governments have not been immune to such concerns and changes, although progress towards a stronger public health response has been seen as dilatory compared to other European countries. (Allsop 1996). That said, during this period, there have been some developments which suggest a more broadly based response to the health needs of the population. This reflects, on the face of it, an acknowledgement that:

1. Attention weighted heavily in favour of secondary and tertiary health care services and responses to illness (acute and chronic), as opposed to the primary health sector and health promotion, is a limited and certainly costly way of meeting the increasing complexity and levels of demand created by the wide health needs of the population.

2. The promotion of the nation's health can only succeed if proper attention is given to the wider environmental, social, political, economic and individual lifestyle determinants of health, together with action to increase people's awareness of their impact on health; and support to challenge and to address any adverse health outcomes.

As Baggott (1994) put it:

The many challenges facing health systems require a much broader approach than simply expanding health services.

Within the UK in the 1990s initial Government concerns and responses have revolved around management and organisational reform, to be closely followed by the creation of a policy for health. By 1992, with the internal market reforms in place, and a managerial style and ethos underpinning all activity, the Government announced its preferred health policy. The White Paper 'The Health of the Nation' (Cmd 1986 1992) set out a strategy which:

> . . . *was to provide us with new opportunities to raise our sights beyond the provision of health care – important though that is – to health itself. The National Health Service was to be at the centre of that strategy, but other organisations, every department in Whitehall, private companies and voluntary bodies, local authorities, health authorities, employers, trade unions, and individuals of every age would need to play their part.*

By the end of 1996, and in a similar vein, the Conservative Government acknowledged that:

> *The successful delivery of health care requires us to see the health service in its wider context. The objective of health policy is not simply to deliver health care, it is to improve the health of the nation. This is why the Government set out clear priorities for improving health in its White Paper 'The Health of the Nation'. The NHS of the future must reflect those priorities. (Cmd 3425 1996)*

In turn then, the Government has put public health and health promotion high on its agenda for the coming years (Cmd 3852 1998):

> *Whilst health generally has improved, far too many people are still falling ill and dying sooner than they should. The National Health Service is there to provide treatment and care when people fall ill – but it is not enough to treat people when they fall ill. We've got to do more to stop them from falling ill in the first place. That means tackling the root causes of the avoidable illnesses. In recent times the emphasis has been on trying to get people to live healthy lives, where necessary by changing their lifestyles. Now we want to see far more attention and Government action concentrated on the things which damage people's health which are beyond the control of the individual, i.e. air pollution, poverty, low wages, unemployment, poor housing, crime and disorder.*

So, will Klein's conclusion to his analysis of the creation of the National Health Service (NHS) in 1948 that: 'Britain had a policy for health services, but not a policy for health' (Klein 1992), continue to hold true as we move into the twenty-first century? Many nurses will be hoping that the apparent continuing shift of focus towards a primary care-led NHS, together with a new agenda for public health, will at long last create a more balanced and effective care agenda in response to the health needs of the population. They will be looking for policy changes which provide ultimately a legitimised context for health care, which combines both health promotion activity together with secondary and tertiary interventions. However, at this relatively early stage of the current Government's life, many nurses will continue to be cautious, and perhaps even a little cynical given their experiences under previous governments. After all, the health strategy of 1992, although presented in glossy and attractive packaging, lacked real detail for action, specific and clear financial backing, and thus in effect any really serious intent (Butler 1997). Rather than providing a positive health policy backcloth to the NHS internal market reforms, it has been described as a figleaf behind which a dismantling of the NHS was slowly taking place, to become an even more limited medical illness service (Fatchett 1994). For many with positive health agendas, like school nurses, community learning disability and mental health nurses and health visitors, role diminution and redundancy have become a reality in recent years (Health Services Journal 1997). In spite of positive claims to the contrary, a health promotional framework for NHS activity has remained a relative side-show to other more pressing policy imperatives around the vagaries, failures, and continuing emphasis on illness services.

This chapter will develop a discussion around some of the issues raised so far, and not least on the future likelihood of a serious public health focus for the NHS under a Labour Government. The chapter will be broken up into the following sections:

1. The concept of health – Defining a focus for care.
2. The promotion of health and health service changes – A consideration of those aspects which have or have not provided a health promotional framework for activities to address the wider determinants of health.
3. The Health of the Nation – the Green Paper (Cmd 1523 1991).
4. The Health of the Nation – the White Paper (Cmd 1986 1992) – To clarify the previous Government's perspective on health and the expected role of the NHS in the field of health promotion.
5. The Labour Government: an agenda for health – The potential for the public health and primary care sectors to become central foci for health care delivery in the future.

THE CONCEPT OF HEALTH

Definitions of the concept of health are wide ranging, multifaceted and personal. Health may be viewed as absence of disease on one hand, as well-being on the other, or even something involving personal capacity or resources for living (Cribb 1993). Many terms also are used to denote something other than health: ill health, sickness, disease, illness, disability, handicap, impairment. The multiple foci of writing and research about health and illness clearly reflect the different and differing perception held by professionals, politicians and the public alike.

The medical model of health

The dominant health model which has been powerfully supported over time is that created by the medical profession. This is unsurprising as they have been seen as the perceived experts on health and health care because of their greater knowledge and skills than other professionals.

> *Stereotypically, the medical model can be viewed as thinking of man as a machine. Man is healthy when the human is in perfect working order, thus the engineering model. By tinkering around with the individual pieces (organs) the machine (man) can be repaired to function appropriately.*
> *(Long 1984)*

Important parts of this model are that ill health is seen as a natural and bio-logical breakdown of the body, and, as ill health befalls individuals, it is they who need to be cured or given care. It is unsurprising then that people have likened the NHS to 'a garage for putting faulty human bodies back on the road again' (Klein 1992). The wider environmental determinants of ill health, or health for that matter, are not in the 'engineering' model a primary con-sideration. The focus of diagnosis and cure is on the disease and its process, and so, for example, surgery will be used to remove a cancer, or drugs prescribed to relieve depression. Other wider health promotional activity around these issues would be seen as beyond the medical model remit, so thus limiting or even ignoring the finding or eradication of the social root causes.

The social model of health

An opposing perception of health is one that views it as a concept with social origins. It has been referred to as having an ecological or environmental basis. It is demonstrated via the new public health approaches of recent years, and is concerned with the wider determinants of health – lifestyles, health services, economic policies and unemployment. As Goodwin explained:

> *Like the "old" public health, expounded by people like Florence Nightingale, and her Victorian medical officer of health contemporaries, the new public health is about environmental and personal health protection. But it goes much further to call for explicit public policies which will as the World*

Health Organization puts it, make the healthy choices of behaviour and life-styles the easier choices. (Goodwin 1992)

Many as we all know have argued that greater levels of health and wellness are a result of better standards of living, and not necessarily because of our nursing and medical health services.

The appraisal of influences on health in the past suggests that we owe the improvement, not to what happens when we are ill, but to the fact that we do not often become ill, and we remain well, not because of specific measures such as vaccination and immunisation, but because we enjoy a higher standard of nutrition and live in a healthier environment. (McKeown 1976)

The social model of health thus pushes attention and activity towards an emphasis on finding out why ill health occurs, a greater concern for care over cure, and a shift towards an environmental or public health approach.

A nurse model of health

Nurses in reality may well use a mix of the above health models as their guiding philosophy for care, perhaps stressing one side more than another depending upon their role and situation. In any event, it would be invidious and mechanistic to carve out one position or another in holy writ. Individuals need to reflect on their own philosophy of health and equate it to professional and contextual remits, with a good understanding of the real health issues faced by the population. As Cribb says:

We cannot solve the problems of health care by fastening upon a definition of health. Some of the time it is helpful to use a conception of health which concentrates on specific measurable objectives; some of the time it is helpful to be reminded of the infinite variety of elements that can contribute to life's quality; and it is always helpful to remember that health care involves enabling individuals to function well as people and not just as biological organisms. (Cribb 1993)

In nursing education a commonly used definition of health has been that of the World Health Organization (WHO) in 1946 – a state of complete physical, mental and social well-being, not merely the absence of disease or infirmity (WHO 1946). However, this has been criticised because it describes an ideal state which is unrealistic. Others now look to perhaps more acceptable definitions of health which offer us some sort of realisable objective. We might consider that of the Ottawa Charter for Health (WHO 1986b):

Health is created and lived by people within the settings of their everyday life; where they learn, work, play and love. Health is created by caring for oneself and others, by being able to take decisions and have control over one's life circumstances, and by ensuring that the society one lives in creates conditions that allow the attainment of health by all its members.

This definition is wide ranging, embracing not only the prevention of ill health, but also the promotion of health. It clearly represents 'an attempt to move from planning medical care services to planning for healthy people and healthy environments' (Luker and Orr 1992).

This perspective on health is in line with the goal of the WHO of health for all by the year 2000 (WHO 1978, 1981, 1985):

The main social target of WHO in the coming decades should be the attainment by all citizens of the world by the year 2000 of a level of health that will permit them to lead a socially and economically productive life.

The UK Government was a signatory to the 1984 agreement to work towards the 38 health for all targets set out for countries in the European region of WHO (WHO 1984, 1986a). It is worth noting at this point that the then Health Secretary, Virginia Bottomley, said she viewed 'The Health of the Nation' strategy as keeping in line with WHO's aims and objectives. She said that these would be built on 'in a way designed to meet the particular cir-cumstances in this country' (Cmd 1986 1992). Presumably she was linking the health strategy with that of the NHS reforms and wider Government and social and economic policy. The NHS would be expected to make its contri-bution in healthy alliance with all of the other interested players, as set out in the White Paper.

A healthy future for health promotion

At this point then, in the early 1990s, we might well have concluded that the Conservative Government's health policy intentions reflected a broad defini-tion of health, and a wide-ranging goal covering all levels of intervention – primary, secondary and tertiary. It appeared to offer the potential to develop roles in primary care practice and to ensure as they stated in the White Paper (Cmd 1986 1992), '. . . further continuing improvements in the health of the nation . . .', and the provision of '. . . even better health care for the millions of people who rely on the National Health Service'.

But was this a new departure in reality from what had been before? For most of the twentieth century health policy had been more concerned with the provision of hospital services than with health promotion. Was it possible that the scope of practice for NHS nurses was to be radically developed? Had a new enthusiasm for public health initiatives swept over the Government, perhaps because of a sudden recognition that the complexity of health issues in a developed society required something more than the promotion, finance and provision of health care services? Or, were there more covertly functional or ideological forces at play? Rather than widening the agenda for nurses, was the real intention to reduce the remit of the NHS's responsibility for health, and that of the professionals within it? In this way, the work involved in health promotion activity was passed onto other agencies and individuals. Indeed, a look back at trends in health policy direction, especially from the early 1980s onwards, tends to support the view that a public health response from Government has always taken second place to that of the provision of hospital and illness services. While often giving the impression of changing the focus and emphasis, in practice this has not been achieved. For example, the title of the White Paper setting out the NHS reforms in 1989, 'Working for Patients' (Cmd 555 1989) was semantically appropriate. It was concerned in the main with hospital services and patients, as its contents make clear. As such the title meant what it said. It is evident that a health policy package around promoting the public's health, something like in the nineteenth century, is still waiting for its time to come again. It therefore remains to be seen whether the appointment by the Labour Government of a specific Minister of Public Health will realise just that opportunity in the future. However, before considering the potential for a significant change in emphasis from health care to public health, it is worthwhile reminding ourselves of previous health policy developments, all also apparently aimed at promoting the nation's health.

THE PROMOTION OF HEALTH AND HEALTH SERVICE CHANGES

The promotion of the nation's health is not a late twentieth century idea. Progress had already been made even before the well-reported sanitary revolution of the nineteenth century. Quarantine facilities and basic programmes to care for the sick were already in evidence. However, the upheavals of the industrial revolution and the creation of immense social problems provided the impetus for a more developed collective approach to the public's health, with the provision over time of clean water, sewerage systems, street lighting, better housing and immunisation. If industry and thus the economic base of the country were to be thriving and healthy, it was imperative that those who worked to make it happen were fit to play their part. As the Royal Sanitary Commission stated in 1871:

> *The constant relation between the health and vigour of the people and the welfare and commercial prosperity of the state requires no argument . . . public health is public wealth. (Acheson 1988)*

It was therefore increasingly accepted by succeeding governments during the nineteenth and early twentieth century, that there was a need for government to intervene to enhance individual efforts to be healthy. Without a doubt, the 40% rejection on medical grounds of applicants who wished to be recruited for active service in the Boer War helped to initiate the subsequent governmental interventions in health care. The 1919 Health Act charged the Minister of Health to take all such steps as may be desirable to secure the preparation, effective carrying out and coordination of measures conducive to the health of the people.

Prevention of illness and the promotion of health were clearly of great importance, and activity ranged widely. We see the creation of infectious disease hospitals, new general hospitals, and special services for pregnant women, mothers, babies and school children. The Minister was also extensively involved in the control of those wider environmental factors along with housing and food hygiene which, it was accepted, all affected the health of the population. At this stage then, the determinants of health were seen as complex, multifaceted and as such were the remit and responsibility of the Health Minister and his department.

The Second World War raised questions about all previous government policy, and provided the catalyst for the new post-war creation of the Welfare State. A collective response to those issues was accepted as a necessary role of government. People needed to be helped to health, particularly in the control of those factors over which they could exercise little power. For example, the unemployment of the 1930s and the resultant poverty and ill health were factors which only the development of a healthy economic and industrial base could heal.

The Beveridge plan (Beveridge 1942), to fight the so-called giants of want, ignorance, disease, idleness and squalor, provided a post-war strategy to shape and to control those powerful determinants of the public's health. Financial benefits, state education, public housing initiatives, employment creation and development, and a health service were collective responses to meet the needs of the population. All were aimed to help individuals to be healthy, and to create in turn a healthy nation.

In spite of much popular support for such developments, the post-war Labour Government had to fight tooth and nail to carry through their proposed legislation. The NHS Bill faced, as we already know, strong opposition from many members of the medical profession (Foot 1973). Aneurin Bevan was forced to make political concessions to this very powerful professional group but, nonetheless, carried the Bill through to enactment, and thereby delivered a national health service to this country.

The new NHS of 1948 was not only to provide medical care, but to:

◆ provide an equitable distribution of health care services;
◆ provide services which were accountable to the nation;

◆ give a sense of collective purpose or mission; and importantly
◆ promote the health of the nation.

Along with the other structures of the Welfare State, the health service would be part of a great collective enterprise made up of several branches across Government, all helping individuals to be healthy.

That said, the focus for professional health care was from that point onward to be shaped by, and pulled into, a narrower and increasingly powerful hospital and medically defined illness framework. It was a situation which would continue during the decades to follow. Public health, primary care and general practice were to be sidelined and clearly seen as second best, at the side of the ever-developing and powerful hospital sector. During the 1950s and 1960s primary health care acquired a Cinderella-like reputation, reflecting not least the disproportionate amount of NHS funds spent on increasingly expensive hospital treatments and buildings. However, by the early 1970s those with primary health care interests begin to see some shifting of focus in their favour in government health policy activities.

The 1970s – A new look at primary health care and a health agenda

This decade witnessed a period of economic crisis, and successive governments were forced to examine and to re-address their levels of public expenditure. Orthodoxy determined that efforts be made to reduce public spending, and at the same time to create new ways of providing public services, like health care, in a politically acceptable, and more cost-effective way than hitherto.

As Baggott (1994) says:

> . . . there was an increasing recognition, that the burden of illness in modern societies required something more than a narrow medicalised response. The invigoration of the primary care setting, together with a new agenda for health, seemed to offer the Government a way forward.

Initial discussion revolved around the need for each individual to take responsibility for his own health, and to play a part in preventing the rising levels of heart disease, accidents, alcoholism, mental illness, smoking, diet and drug-related diseases. (Department of Health and Social Security 1976a). However, the White Paper which followed – 'Prevention and Health' (Cmd 7047 1977) – appeared fairly half-hearted about making new health and primary care focused moves. While it demonstrated the Government's interest in a strategy for improving public health, it did not appear to want to shift resources into agendas outside the curative hospital settings.

By 1979, and with the election of a new Conservative government, previous unwillingness to challenge and to change the powerful and increasingly costly hospital sector was put aside. The new Government believed that the primary health care sector based around general practice had the potential (if reformed and sharpened) to reduce the ever-rising cost of hospital services.

Developments in the 1980s – initial themes

The continuing need, and indeed the desire to reduce public expenditure across all the boundaries of welfare state provision including health care, was the prime motive for change during this decade. While a more business-like and competitive environment was created in the NHS as a whole, at the same time, users and potential users were to be encouraged more strongly than ever before to take greater individual responsibility for their own health – an emphasis which fitted in well with the ideological approach of New Right conservatism. Health education and promotion, now the concern of all nurses and other health practitioners, were to provide the population with sufficient information and advice on the pursuit of healthy lifestyles. It was then up to individuals to make their own health choices (to stand on their own two feet), particularly in regard to diet, exercise, smoking, sexual activity and alcohol.

Around this time, the publication of the Black Report (Black 1980) provided research evidence to show that there was a link between inequalities in income and other resources and poor health. However, it failed to change the Government's belief that individuals could change their lifestyles for the better if they wished, and, given enough information. As such each person was seen as ultimately totally responsible for their own health status. The wider determinants of health as proposed in Black's findings were believed to be the responsibility of individuals, and not Government. This of course is the opposite position to that taken by the nineteenth century politicians, and the post-war Labour Government, who believed that people needed to be helped to health, as well as helping themselves.

During the decade, increasing Government interest in reducing public expenditure, and in providing more effective and cost-efficient health care, resulted in a change of apparent focus for health care delivery. As already noted, general practice and the primary health care team became an area of growing favour (Cmd 249 1987). Primary care based on general practice teams was seen as less costly than hospital care, and provided an opportunity (if its 'gatekeeper' role was sharpened up) to reduce public expenditure. A new contract of employment for GPs (Department of Health 1989b) now included the requirement to provide health promotion and disease prevention services alongside secondary and tertiary services.

The apparent empowerment of general practice at this stage, and support for a more positive health agenda than hitherto, was, on the face of it, suggestive of a fresh look by Government in response to the developing health problems in the UK of the 1980s (National Audit Office (NAO) 1989). However, while the trend towards a more health promotional agenda was in the right direction, others have reached the conclusion that the response was both ideologically and economically driven and reflected other goals (Soothill, Henry & Kendrick 1992, Gough, Maslin-Prothero & Masterton 1994, Hart 1994). The intended impact of the underpinning reforms of both management and structure of the NHS during this period was to limit rather than to expand NHS responsibility and expenditure. The extra attention given to general practice and primary prevention activity was a means to another end – to reduce costs, activity and professional power implicit within the hospital sector. A serious move towards a primary care approach involved a great deal more than the negative impetus behind the Government's apparent motives.

Ashton & Seymour (1988), for example, outlined the facets of primary care which WHO had included in its definition of the concept in practice (WHO 1978). These included:

◆ The promotion of self-help.
◆ The integration of medical/nursing care with other care sectors.
◆ Environmental improvements.
◆ The promotion of good health rather than the promotion of simply good health services.
◆ Attempts to meet the needs of under-privileged and under-serviced groups.
◆ Encouragement of wider community participation in the planning and delivery of health services.

By contrast, it is interesting to note the limited application of the concept of primary care made by the Government. On the one hand, it had encouraged health promotion and self-care, but in reality, on the other, it appeared disinterested in the negative impacts on people's lives, and not just those people who had the least resources. The Government promoted individual consumer choice and consumerism in health care, but it was apparently not that interested in any collective response to meeting health need, like community participation projects. It appeared also to fail to recognise the formal and informal care roles of other professionals, agencies and individuals working outside of the NHS. As Baggott (1994) described it:

> . . . *the government's primary care reforms have concentrated on the NHS, and in particular on the family practitioner services, as the principal means for improving primary care.*

So, in spite of protestations to the contrary by the Government, this supposed support for a broad primary health care agenda apparently ignored WHO's view that:

> *. . . the key to solving many health problems lies outside the health sector, or is in the hands of people themselves – in order to meet contemporary challenges to health, it is necessary for all elements of society to contribute.*
> *(WHO 1978)*

At this stage stress was continuing to be laid on secondary and tertiary interventions at the expense of a true primary health care approach. As such, the NHS, and indeed general practice within it, was to continue to be perceived by many as an illness service, or as noted earlier, as 'a garage for putting faulty human bodies back on the road again'. The promotion of health appeared to be a side-line in the developing business of NHS care provision. That said, no one should be too surprised. After all, high-tech medical interventions in a hospital setting have, over time, been perceived by the public, health professionals and politicians alike as evidence and proof of a successful health service, fit for a highly developed society and nation. Forty years of NHS policy which have reflected this stance have left a structure, organisation and a culture within the NHS which still reflect old roots that are illness based and focused on medicine.

So, would the internal market reforms of the 1990s lead to the creation of a policy for health and a broader primary health care agenda for the NHS?

The NHS post 1989 – illness or health promoter?

The first review of the NHS for 40 years (Cmd 555 1989) coupled with that of community care (CMD 849 1989) led, as we know, to the enactment of the NHS and Community Care Act in June 1990. The reforms, involving profound changes in structure, organisation and management of the NHS have, it is suggested, enabled the Government 'to focus on health as much as health care'. That said, the Government's review of the fault-strewn old NHS was perceived by many as an examination of only one part of the total health care picture in the UK. By definition, how could it be anything else? The assessment of the NHS and its workings was not concerned with exploring the potential of the ongoing wider fringe health care activity, least of all that which blurred with what was to be termed 'social care' and social issues. The review was about hospitals, general practice and ill people, and not about a positive health agenda and all that this implies. In this way, the review only provided at best a partial diagnosis and thus a partial prescription for improving health care provision. It really cannot be seen as even trying to meet the wide and complex health care issues of UK society today. As Harrison et al (1989) said, 'The diagnosis it can be argued, is rather narrow and pays scant regard to wider issues including the persistence of health inequalities, the level of preventable illness, and alleged underfunding of the NHS which prompted the review in the first place.' Others have argued that the White

Paper continued 'to see the NHS as a national hospital service with its title – Working For Patients – reflecting a lack of commitment to health promotion and preventive medicine' (Community Outlook 1989).

Goodwin believed the White Paper was not 'much interested in health as such; health promotion was only mentioned once in passing as one of the responsibilities of health authorities, with no clue as to how that responsibility would be expressed in service terms' (Goodwin 1989b). The Association of Community Health Councils (ACHCEW 1989) noted that the White Paper was orientated almost entirely to the acute sector, and that huge sections of the NHS were omitted or dealt with cursorily. Community care was not discussed, and public health referred to only briefly. The RCN said the Government in its review 'was looking up the wrong end of a telescope, and should be concentrating its attention not on acute care, but on services for the large and rising numbers of elderly people and on the promotion of good health' (Editorial 1989).

Grave doubts were expressed early on about the review's findings and solutions. Not only in more general terms was the document perceived as lacking in detail concerning the proposed changes, and as a threat to the long-term viability of the principles underlying a national health service – but it also appeared isolationist in its exclusivity of emphasis on hospital and medical services. It also presented a limited view of the concept of health and the role of nurses (particularly community nurses), who would have expected to be mentioned more widely.

Community nurses' concerns

The continuing emphasis on the medical and curative aspects is exemplified by the persistent support of the model for health care for people outside hospital which concentrates on the GP as first point of contact. This is totally in line of course with the trend of general practice empowerment and development following the 1987 White Paper (Fatchett 1989, 1990). The opportunity for community nurses to take a different and truly primary health care approach to care as proposed in the Cumberlege Report (Department of Health and Social Security 1986), was rejected by the Government. With the GP as the first point of contact, health interventions invariably become secondary and tertiary. Others of course will disagree, looking to the health promotional aspects of the GP contract. In order to show that positive health approaches are indeed supported, they look to those nurses in general practice who, they claim, now have unlimited opportunity for enormous creativity in their primary health care role. Health visitors, district nurses and many others also, similarly carry out a wide variety of well-reported health promotional activity on behalf of their employer bodies.

However, if community nurses were so important in delivering the

Government's positive health strategy, why did they only merit a single line in the White Paper? District nurses and health visitors (and what about all the other community nurses?) were seen as needed to be provided locally 'on grounds of practicality', and health promotion was only referred to in passing as one of the responsibilities of health authorities. So much then for acknowledgement of the enormous amount of effective primary health care work that has been, and is being carried out by nurses in the community. One might be forgiven for describing it as dismissive.

Health–social care split

Another concern expressed at the time of publication of the White Paper was that no response or reference to the Griffiths' Report on Community Care (Griffiths 1988) was made. Accusations flew around, and dismay was expressed because the NHS appeared to be equated with hospital services and general practice. The total focus appeared to be on illness and treatment, and other levels of caring and states of wellness were ignored. Large groups in the population (e.g. the elderly, the mentally handicapped, the disabled) appeared to be off the agenda, but who clearly did receive care from NHS nurses and other care professionals. No true positive health agenda was addressed because presumably it was not seen as NHS business. Both health care and health appeared to be defined tightly (although no explicit definitions were given), and effectively the role of nurses was made leaner. Indeed, the publication of the Government's Community Care White Paper 'Caring for People,' (Cmd 849 1989) only confirmed fears that health care was indeed being redefined and its remit slimmed down. Social care was to become the responsibility of local authorities and social carers.

It is little wonder then that community nurses in particular began to express discomfort at that stage, not only for their professional survival, but as health promoters concerned with the multiplicity of determinants of health. They felt their activities were being compromised and potential role enrichment disappearing. The unnatural split being created between health (health authority) and social care (local authority) concerns appeared to challenge their holistic nursing approach to work. Their employing health authorities, with an eye on budgets, were very likely to define how far their work could merge and cross with local authority social care provision.

Indeed, the expressed wish of the Government was to ensure that 'nurses' time was deployed to best effect on work which required special skills, leaving work which did not require those skills to be done by others'. This reflects, as we will see in a later chapter, the early dissection and paring down of the professional role of the nurse by others, who in turn, fail to understand that nursing care is about much more than providing technical skills and acting as assistants to doctors. Nurses are concerned with all the realities of people's lives, not just those tasks which can be easily qualified, quantified and costed. Unfortunately, the changes presented in both the NHS and Community Care reform White Papers reinforced a medicalised concept of health and health care, and this underpinned what the role of the nurse was to be within the reforming NHS. This in turn served to create in reality a fragmentation of care by nurses and perhaps a reduction in standards for those who received that care.

Fragmentation or integration of care?

It is worth noting that health policy analysts have described the creation of this organisational split in delivering health and social care as a profound turning point in NHS history. According to Holliday (1992), the earlier 1974 NHS reorganisation was a change based on a theme of organisational integration, bringing together those strands of health care provision which had been split in a tripartite fashion in 1948 when the NHS began. The aim in 1974 was to bring together primary, hospital and community care services to improve health care planning and organisation and thus to improve further the nation's health.

It is somewhat strange then to see a new 1990 fragmentation of care provision with the emergence of hospital and community trusts, directly managed units, budget holding general practices, new local authority responsibilities, and the increasing promotion of private and voluntary sector involvement. In effect, the new health and social care internal market structures have surely created fragmented rather than integrated means of meeting the health needs of the population. Whether or not this promoted multidisciplinary collaboration and provided the smooth and seamless care so promised is debatable, and will be discussed in another chapter. However, if we doubt the method and process set up to promote the nation's health at this stage, we must accept that there was a potential threat to achieving healthy outcomes:

> *For patients and clients . . . the threat can be simply stated – the major risk for them lies in the inevitable fragmentation of care into easy-to-cost units which bear no relationship to the continuity of human lives, in sickness or in health. (Goodwin 1989a)*

So far then we have observed the apparent focus of the health reforms on the hospital and medical services, coupled with the virtual disregard for community care, and the limited mention of public health. Sadly, this perhaps represented a belief that they were not to be aspects central to health care provision, or indeed to the conceptual framework for health promotion embodied within NHS provision. The apparent emphasis appeared to be on directing resources to services for ill people, rather than at health promotional activity. In response to that final accusation, however, others will refer us to the promised remit for the district health authorities. As the White Paper said:

> *DHAs can . . . concentrate on ensuring that the health needs of the population for which they are responsible are met; that there are effective services for the prevention and control of diseases and the promotion of health; that their population has access to a comprehensive range of high quality, value for money services. (Cmd 555 1989)*

All of the above did sound an optimistic note. However, we need to reflect on the fact that no definitions of either 'health' or 'need' were provided in the White Paper, and thus the purpose of the NHS in general, and DHAs in this particular instance were unclear and ill-defined.

The DHAs of course had the opportunity to tackle persistent environmentally and socially induced health problems in their authority areas, and thus to provide a very welcome response. They could also wear their strictly 'market hats' and pursue narrow non-risk-taking approaches with an eye to budget balances and contract making. In the light of experience at this stage, it would seem that the latter scenario was the more likely. DHAs like local authorities implementing community care reforms have had to bow to the realities of resources available both in terms of finance and services when making assessments of need. Cost-conscious purchasers cannot afford to take risks when their own employment contracts are on the line, and so the temptation is surely to take the well-trodden paths of mainstream health care activity. It has always been easier to quantify physical/medical interventions than to measure activities with potentially immeasurable outcomes. You only have to ask any health visitor about some of their resourcing difficulties for health education and promotion activities, in particular with work concerned with child protection, the homeless, travellers, prostitutes, indeed in any less than mainstream health care fields.

At this point we might conclude that the NHS Review and subsequent Act created new market-like structures, business-like aims and objectives, and further reinforced the limited medicalised concept of health which had underpinned much NHS activity over time. Far from opening up into the wider fields of social and environmental health, the NHS appeared to be pulled back even more than ever into a medical and illness service. While some of the descriptive language in the White Paper emphasised the opposite, the detail within it, and the subsequent Working Papers (Department of Health 1989a), probably provided a truer picture of policy intentions. Doctors, medical services and hospitals were placed centre stage, with nurses and a wider health agenda essentially ignored. Within the NHS, nurses as health promoters were to be potentially limited in those aspects which would be perceived as within their health care roles. It is against this particular backcloth that 'The Health of the Nation' strategy must be examined. It seems already impossible to imagine that the newly emerging NHS was to be in any way fit enough to meet that particular role.

'THE HEALTH OF THE NATION' – THE GREEN PAPER (CMD 1523 1991)

Having introduced its controversial health service reforms, the Government, according to many critics, published its Green Paper on health to divert attention towards more positive discussion. According to William Waldegrave, the then Secretary of State for Health, it was:

> *The first time that an explicit health strategy has been proposed for England. At its heart is the proposal to set challenging health objectives and targets to improve the overall health of the nation. Their scope reflects the fact that my task as Secretary of State is to focus on better health just as much as on better health care. The Green Paper enshrines that wider health objective. I am happy to tell the House that our approach has been endorsed in warm terms by the World Health Organization whose Health for All by the year 2000 programme started the production of such strategies world-wide. (Waldegrave 1991)*

So while the earlier reforms laid emphasis on mechanisms, and means rather than ends, attention was now to be focused on improvements in health. A very consensual approach appeared to be taken by involving and inviting as much opinion as possible to discuss the paper's contents, unlike in the case of the NHS Review. However, criticism still came.

Many were pleased to see an acknowledgement of the multiplicity of determinants of health 'from genetic inheritance, through personal behaviour, family and social circumstances to the physical and social environment' (Delamothe 1991). But for others, the Green Paper failed to recognise the importance of poverty as a cause of poor health and to recommend targets for its reduction, (Carlisle 1991, Hodges 1991). It failed to acknowledge the importance of unemployment and poor housing. It did not address the issue of health inequalities. It lacked a commitment to sufficient funding. Insufficient weight was placed on the role of government departments other than the Department of Health. Indeed doubts were expressed as to the commitment of the Government as a whole. It was also seen as placing too much emphasis on the role of individual action and not enough on collective action.

Clearly, there were supporters who viewed it as a potential opportunity for the NHS to be moved towards a new health agenda rather than remaining an illness-focused service. Others in response expressed more cynical feelings as to the Government's true intentions. Having felt profoundly challenged by the

NHS review, and being somewhat unbelieving as to the promises about the necessary level of resourcing for the NHS, it was clearly hard for some to believe that the Government was taking the health agenda seriously. It did little to reassure sceptics that on the very day that the Green Paper was launched in the House of Commons, Conservative MEPs were vetoing a proposed ban on tobacco advertising throughout Europe (Carlisle 1991). So, while on the one hand demonstrating some awareness of the need for a collective response by Government in promoting the people's health, it failed to follow through some of its own ideas and it provided a partial response only. For example, as one commentator said:

> *The food safety and diet targets do not extend to changing government policy nutritional guidelines for schools or for an integrated food and agriculture policy. They ignore the clear evidence that the difference in income between the rich and poor is the major determinant of a nation's health. Instead the targets are centred around individual behaviour and specific disease. (Scott-Samuel 1991)*

It was inevitable, and perhaps understandable, that many in the nursing and medical media criticised the contents fully.

'THE HEALTH OF THE NATION' – THE WHITE PAPER (CMD 1986 1992)

The publication of the White Paper response in July 1992 was slightly delayed because of the intervening April General Election. The White Paper was, according to Virginia Bottomley, a landmark for the NHS and the next logical step in health care reforms. As she explained, 'now that the structural and management reforms were in place, it was time to work on a policy for health' (Bottomley 1992).

Many commentators welcomed the new stress on promoting health, and although acknowledging the obvious importance of working at the five selected areas for action, were disappointed that the emphasis was on preventing specific illnesses rather than on promoting health. Again, and unsurprisingly, great concern was expressed at the failure to address the issues of poverty, inequality, unemployment and poor housing. As one said: 'The Government has set simplistic targets, but they do not address the underlying issues. Poverty and deprivation are important factors in ill-health. Mrs Bottomley has floated a few ideas but you could hardly call it a strategy – it's largely window dressing.' (Kearney 1992).

The Health Visitors' Association (HVA) for example, pointed out that studies clearly demonstrated links between poverty and children's health, and Buttigieg expressed her fears that 'it was hard to see how this White Paper will bring real help to families struggling to raise healthy children in substandard housing with barely enough money to feed them through the week' (Buttigieg 1992). Other criticisms included the document's emphasis on individual as opposed to collective action, and with this, a lack of belief that sufficient funding would be forthcoming to carry out the work needed as, 'the intention is to focus resources' already given to the NHS. (Carlisle 1992).

One issue which pervaded much of the White Paper discussion was that of smoking and the lack of a ban on tobacco advertising. As Chambers, Killoran & McNeill (1991) had pointed out the year before:

> *Glamorous images of smoking portrayed by the industry undermine the influence of health education in schools, and help to create the view that smoking is adult and socially acceptable. If the Government is serious about achieving the smoking targets and protecting children from the promotion of cigarettes it should support a ban.*

On leaving office in 1997, the Conservative Government was still relying on price, education, self-control and reviews on the role of advertising as a means of achieving their health targets on smoking.

SOME CONCLUDING THOUGHTS ON THE CONSERVATIVE ADMINISTRATION'S RESPONSES TO HEALTH NEED

The NHS changes since 1979 appear to have laid emphasis on the medical–illness aspects of care, in spite of assertions to the contrary. The concept of health underpinning both professional care and thus health promotion has been redefined. The health promotion strategy outlined in the White Paper chose targets which were illness focused, and appeared to offload the responsibility of controlling the wider social determinants of health onto others, many of whom do not work under the umbrella of the NHS.

While accepting then that health promotion activity belongs to many other arenas also, 'The Health of the Nation' strategy could never bring about all the improvements it said it wanted, without a commitment from all other government departments to tackle the wider issues of poverty. As Buttigieg (1993) said:

> *To make real progress we need an economy based on employment, proper childcare, good housing and support for single parents. In the end those are the gaps in the Health of the Nation.*

Indeed, if we consider all the activity during the period of four Conservative administrations to reduce still further the Welfare State provision derived from invalidity and other benefits, and the persistence of high unemployment, it is easy to see that many individuals have probably found it more and more difficult to take decisions and to have control over their own life circumstances. A large group of such people are now by all accounts still needing to be 'helped to health' (Brindle1997, Chadda 1998).

The previous Government's health strategies for the NHS appeared then to be limited in focus. Furthermore, in practice, it was also going to be difficult for other government departments, under pressure in their own spending areas, to come to the rescue or even to the support of the Department of Health. A broad view of health promotion requires collaboration across all government departments: a Whitehall obsessed with spending cuts was never likely to provide an appropriate context. The strategy for the promotion of 'The Health of the Nation' became in reality a side-show to wider changes taking place both within and without the NHS during the past decade and a half.

So, what does the future hold for a new health policy under a Labour Government? Will its health programme provide a more successful way forward?

THE LABOUR GOVERNMENT: AN AGENDA FOR HEALTH

In February 1998, the Government published its consultative Green Paper on public health called 'Our Healthier Nation' (Cmd 3852 1998). It proposed two main aims:

1. To improve the health of the population as a whole, by increasing the length of people's lives and the number of years people spend free from illness.
2. To improve the health of the worst off in society and to narrow the health gap.

In order to fulfil these important aims, the Public Health Minister announced that a new approach to health was being proposed. The Government wished to pursue a 'third way', 'between the old extremes of individual victim blaming on the one hand, and nanny state social engineering on the other'. This third way involved the creation of a national contract for better health. Under this contract, the Government, local communities and individuals would need to join in partnership to improve the nation's health. This involved a number of important contributions:

◆ The Government will help assess the risk to health, and provide information to people which is accurate, understandable and credible.
◆ Health authorities will have a key role in leading local alliances to develop health improvement programmes.

◆ Local authorities will have a new duty to promote the economic, social and environmental well-being of the area.

◆ Businesses will be responsible for improving the health and safety of their own employees.

◆ Voluntary bodies are to act as advocates to give a powerful voice to local people.

◆ Individuals are to take responsibility for their own health.

To focus and to develop the health contract in a structured way, three settings for action were set out:

1. Healthy schools – focusing on children.
2. Healthy workplaces – focusing on adults.
3. Healthy neighbourhoods – focusing on older people.

In this way, attention would be given across the age range, from childhood to older adulthood. According to Reid (1998):

> *If individuals do their bit by following a healthy lifestyle, employers promote healthier workforces, and the NHS and town halls provide more equal services and better housing, the Government will tackle unemployment and other causes of social exclusion.*

At the same time, four priority illness areas had been selected for action, setting clear targets for improvement in each area by the year 2010:

1. Heart disease and stroke.
2. Accidents.
3. Cancer.
4. Mental health.

It was argued that rather than have the longer list of ill health reduction targets as in 'The health of the Nation' (Cmd 1986 1992), this strategy could be simplified. In this way all local health care agencies would be encouraged to set their own targets, reflecting more specifically the assessed health needs of their localities.

The main underpinning theme of this 'third way' approach to improve public health, was a reduction in the health inequality gap between the rich and poor. As Boseley (1998) commented:

> *It pledged to tackle the big social issues – poverty, bad housing, unemployment and other forms of deprivation, that it acknowledges to be at the root of inequalities in health.*

Indeed, the Public Health Minister has said that:

> *... the aim is to improve the health of the most deprived at a rate faster than the overall national rate of improvement in health.*

To achieve this, and indeed all of the aims noted already, will involve the creation of a variety of local, multidisciplinary initiatives, including health living centres, health improvement programmes and health action zones, to name but a few. The details of such developments will take time to emerge, and presently are in the process of creation and development.

All in all, this proposed programme for a new public health agenda is the first government health strategy document to acknowledge a link between poverty and ill health. It also promises a broad and pan-governmental department response. Indeed there is already a cabinet committee representing 12 departments to improve coordination. In addition, some actions, albeit small, have already been taken to combat the social causes of ill health. These include:

◆ A modest increase in housing investment.
◆ The launch of the social exclusion unit.
◆ More opportunity for work as a result of the welfare to work programmes (Editorial 1998).

While these initial moves are positive, the details of this proposed new public health agenda still clearly remain to be fleshed out, and indeed await legislation. The delivery of such a health programme would be welcomed by many, not least because of the breadth of vision for health action offered by the programme. As Reid (1998) concluded:

For the moment, we can afford to applaud because this first shot fired by the Government is in a new and exciting direction. It remains to be seen how far it will be possible to travel along that path.

CONCLUSION

At the beginning of this discussion an argument was made around the need for a UK Government to pursue a more broadly based health agenda than was traditionally the case. An overview of health policy activity in the second half of this century, and specifically over the past two decades, has witnessed significant changes within the NHS, apparently underpinned by a serious commitment to health promotion. The analysis of these developments has however cast doubts upon the argument that the Conservative reforms have led to a coherent and effective health strategy. The Labour Government has now taken up the challenge. They are currently in the process of creating new solutions to the health problems which continue to face the population. The degree to which they achieve success remains to be seen.

Nurses and health visitors meanwhile should take up all opportunities to build 'healthy alliances', to collaborate with other carers of whatever discipline or interest, and to enter into the contract of partnership as proposed by the Government. They should collect evidence of health need and use this to negotiate seriously for NHS resources, both to widen the remit, and to increase the potential for health promotional activity within what appears to have become a more limited and medicalised NHS framework in recent years.

REFERENCES

ACHCEW (Association for Community Health Councils for England and Wales) 1989 Working for Patients? – Response to the Government's review of the NHS. Draft 5. ASCHEW, London

Acheson D 1988 Foreword. Public health in England. Cmd 289. HMSO, London

Allsop J 1996 Health policy and the NHS towards 2000. Longman, London

Ashton J, Seymour H 1988 The new public health. Open University Press, Milton Keynes

Baggott R 1994 Health and health care in Britain. St Martin's Press, London

Beveridge W 1942 Social insurance and allied services. Cmd 6404. HMSO, London

Black D 1980 Inequalities in health: report of a research working group. HMSO, London

Boseley S 1998 Dobson pledges to cut illness gap. The Guardian 6 February, p 10

Bottomley V 1992 Statement on the health of the nation White Paper. HC Debate; c335. Hansard

Brindle D 1997 Fall in life expectancy among the worst off. The Guardian 9 September

Butler P 1997 Green shoots. Health Service Journal 23 October, p 13

Buttigieg M 1992 In: Turner T. A healthy nation. Nursing Times 88(30): 18–19

Buttigieg M 1993 In: Mason P. Healthy living. Nursing Times 89(11): 16–17

Carlisle D 1991 Planning the future. Nursing Times 87(27): 16–17

Carlisle D 1992 Profession is key to White Paper goals. Nursing Times 88(29): 5

Chadda D 1998 Survey confirms health inequalities. Health Service Journal 15 January, p 4

Chambers J, Killoran A, McNeill A 1991 Smoking. British Medical Journal 303: 973–977.

Command 7047 1977 Prevention and Health. HMSO, London

Command 249 1987 Promoting Better Health. HMSO, London

Command 555 1989 Working for Patients. HMSO, London

Command 849 1989 Caring for People. HMSO, London

Command 1523 1991 The Health of the Nation: a consultative document for health in England. HMSO, London

Command 1986 1992 The Health of the Nation: a strategy for health in England. HMSO, London

Command 3425 1996 The National Health Service. A service with ambitions. HMSO, London

Command 3852 1998 Our Healthier Nation. HMSO, London

Community Outlook 1989 Hidden opportunities. Nursing Times March

Cribb A 1993 In: Hinchliff S, Norman S, Schober J (eds) Nursing practice and health care, 2nd edn. Edward Arnold, London

Delamothe T 1991 Health manifestos: the Government. British Medical Journal 302: 1355–1356.

Department of Health 1989a National Health Service review working papers. (Package of 8 booklets.) HMSO, London

Department of Health 1989b General practice in the NHS: the 1990 Contract. HMSO, London

Department of Health and Social Security 1976a Prevention and health: everybody's business. A reassessment of public and personal health. HMSO, London

Department of Health and Social Security 1986 Neighbourhood nursing: a focus for care. Report of the Community Nursing Review. (The Cumberlege Report.) HMSO, London

Editorial 1989 Nursing Times 85(12): 3

Editorial 1998 Prevention is better than cure. The Guardian 6 February, p 18

Fatchett A 1989 Going the way of the dinosaur? Nursing Times 85(27): 59

Fatchett A 1990 Health visiting: a withering profession? Journal of Advanced Nursing 15: 216–222

Fatchett A 1994 Politics, policy and nursing. Baillière Tindall, London

Flynn P 1997 Public health in Europe (employment and social affairs). European Commission, Luxembourg Office

Foot M 1973 Aneurin Bevan, vol 2. Davis Poynter, London

Goodwin S 1989a Storm clouds ahead? Nursing Times 85(10): 44–45

Goodwin S 1989b Looking between the lines of the White Paper. Health Visitor 62(4): 103

Goodwin S 1992 Community nursing and the new public health. Health Visitor 65(3): 78–80

Gough P, Maslin-Prothero S, Masterton A 1994 Nursing and social policy. Butterworth Heinemann, Oxford

Griffiths R 1988 Community care: agenda for action. HMSO, London

Harrison S, Hunter D, Johnston I, Wistow G 1989 Competing for health. A commentary on the NHS review. Nuffield Institute Reports, University of Leeds

Hart C 1994 Behind the mask. Nurses, their unions and nursing policy. Baillière Tindall, London

Health Services Journal 1997 Health visitor cuts would harm child protection. 23 October, p 4

Hodges C 1991 Health of the nation. Nursing Times 87(48): 19

Holliday I 1992 The NHS transformed. Baseline Books, Manchester

Kearney 1992 In: Mihill C. Strategy for improvement or window-dressing. The Guardian 9 July

Klein R 1992 Strengths and frailties of the 1942 citizen's charter. The Guardian 4 March

Long A 1984 Research into health and illness. Gower, London

Luker, K, Orr J 1992 Towards community health nursing. Blackwell Scientific Publications, Oxford

McKeown T 1976 The role of medicine: dream, mirage or nemesis? Nuffield Provincial Hospitals Trust. Oxford University Press, Oxford

National Audit Office (NAO) 1989 Report of the Controller and Auditor General: NHS coronary health. HMSO, London

Reid D 1998 A strategy fit for everyone. The Guardian 11 February, p 6

Scott-Samuel A 1991 In: Carlisle D. Planning the future, Nursing Times 87(27): 16–17

Soothill K, Henry C, Kendrick K 1992 Themes and perspectives in nursing. Chapman and Hall, London

Waldegrave W 1991a Statement on the health of the nation consultative document. HC Debate; C155. Hansard

WHO 1946 Constitution. WHO, Geneva

WHO 1978 Primary health care. WHO, Geneva

WHO 1981 Global strategy for health for all by the year 2000. WHO, Geneva

WHO 1984 Regional strategy for health for all by the year 2000. WHO, Geneva

WHO 1985 Targets for health for all. WHO, Copenhagen

WHO 1986a Nursing and the 38 targets of health for all. A discussion paper. WHO/Euro, Copenhagen

WHO 1986b Ottawa charter for health promotion. Canadian Public Health Association, WHO/Euro, Copenhagen

4

The concept of need

The underpinning rationale for the creation of the National Health Service in 1948 was that of meeting the health needs of the population. The new service was based on the principles of :

◆ Universal availability.
◆ Equality.
◆ Comprehensiveness.

Care was to be provided free at the point of use, and allocated on the basis of individual need. Aneurin Bevan (Minister of Health for the Labour Government in 1945) described the NHS as replacing the fear that many had felt about becoming ill, and having to negotiate the iniquitous market distribution of health care of previous decades. (Bevan 1952) Meeting needs through a publicly funded health service was thus aimed at equalising the opportunity for every citizen to achieve good health, and not just those with sufficient financial resources to meet their needs, whatever the current system of health care distribution.

It is interesting then to consider how the Labour Government of 1948, and all succeeding governments both Conservative and Labour, have claimed to focus the NHS on meeting need. The concept is clearly amenable to different ideological and political interpretations. Perhaps this is not surprising. As O'Keefe, Ottewill, Wall (1994) remind us:

Very difficult choices have to be made in respect of prioritising needs and the deployment of resources to meet them, and no single constituency has the monopoly of wisdom in resolving the moral predicaments to which these choices give rise.

This chapter then will explore further the concept of need, not least because it is a guiding and continuing principle which underpins both health policy and nursing practice within the NHS of today. The following areas will be examined:

1. The concept of need: why look at it?
2. The concept of need: what does it mean?

3. A medical/epidemiological model for needs assessment.
4. An economic model for needs assessment.
5. A social model for needs assessment.
6. The historical usage of the concept of need in health care delivery.
7. The 1980s and 1990s: the reforms and a new perspective on need.
8. The reforms: needs led? Or market led?
9. The future: 'The New NHS. Modern. Dependable'.

THE CONCEPT OF NEED: WHY LOOK AT IT?

All concepts are difficult to define in a scientific and precise way, and every-one will interpret a particular concept within the framework of their own knowledge and experience, to give it both meaning and value. It is perhaps because of this, that the discipline of nursing and its claims to professional status are often challenged. Many of its specific and defining concepts are per-ceived by others as ill-defined, descriptive, common-or-garden words which appear in everyday language. They somehow lack the gravitas of the tradi-tional and classical concepts which surround the medical and legal profes-sions. Words such as caring, helping, supporting, encouraging and empathising suggest a lack of scientific rigour, are subjective, and according to some are so indefinable as to be almost useless. The concept of need also could well be added to this list. According to Bradshaw (1994):

> The concept of need has always been too imprecise, too complex, and too contentious, to be a useful target for policy.

While then the appropriateness and applicability of the concept of need to nursing practice (or indeed the NHS more generally) is open to debate, the notion of meeting need is, and remains for the future, a major underpinning focus for professional nurse care and the health service. (Cmd 3807 1997). As such then, it is a very worthwhile activity to explore both its meaning and usage. It will add to nursing's knowledge base, enhance the ability to explain the concept and nursing's specific concern with it to others. The process will also help highlight alternative explanations, how it is applied in practice, the impact of changing contexts in health care delivery, and the degree to which it has been allowed to focus or to frame the implementation of nursing care overtime. For without a doubt, the interpretations of the concept of need within the NHS environment at any one time will impact on nurse care ini-tiatives – what may or may not be addressed in relation to meeting the assessed needs of clients or patients.

In recent years, for example, statements made by governments around NHS developments have promoted the primacy of the consumer voice, and the importance of meeting expressed needs. In reality of course, as noted in a previous chapter, the apparent development of a consumer-led service has been constrained by the overriding economic perspectives and imperatives of the internal health care market. As Bradshaw reminds us also:

> . . . *the assessment of need has emerged from, and quickly settled into the language of priority setting, economic efficiency, cost effectiveness and the market orientation of the political right. (Bradshaw1994)*

So, while statements have been made applauding successful consumer-led nurse activity in response to need, the reality is that the parameters of nurse care have been defined, constrained and often reduced by the impact of successive Conservative governments' health and economic policy reforms. This observation, incidentally, could well be made about the influence over time of other governments. Interpretations of the concept of need have shifted around over the years, reflecting the ideological and political views of different governments. It seems that as a guiding concept for care it can, to coin a phrase, be all things to all people. Sanderson (1996) refers to it 'as a controversial concept, a subject of dispute, containing conflicting values and interests'. That said, it remains a guiding and underpinning motive for professional nurse care, (United Kingdom Central Council 1992), and as such it should be clarified further. Let us now turn to consider some of the ways in which the concept has been viewed.

THE CONCEPT OF NEED: WHAT DOES IT MEAN?

Initial knowledge gained by many nurses around the concept of need probably links back to teaching on Maslow's hierarchy of needs (Maslow 1954). He theorised on needs which are basic to human growth and development, and which emerge in the following order:

◆ Physiological drives.
◆ Safety.
◆ Love and belongingness.
◆ Esteem needs.
◆ Cognitive needs.
◆ Aesthetic needs.
◆ Self actualisation.

He proposed that once one need was satisfied, another need took over. While a need may not be completely satisfied, it is possible for an individual to move on up through the hierarchy. This Maslovian hierarchy of needs underpinned conceptually many of the nursing models for care which were to be developed in later years. These models aimed to provide a framework for the systematic assessment of health need and the subsequent delivery of appropriately planned and evaluated care. For others who are concerned with the language of need, Bradshaw's 1972 analysis of the concept is often taken as the starting point. His analysis was based on the work for a Masters thesis in the 1970s, in which he sought to clarify what the word need meant when applied to the social needs of people aged 80 and over. The well-reported taxonomy of need he produced is set out below:

1. *Normative need* is defined by experts, professionals, doctors, policy makers, and so on. Often a desirable standard is laid down and compared with the standard that actually exists.
2. *Felt need* is want, desire or subjective views of need which may or may not become expressed need.
3. *Expressed need* is demand or felt need turned into action.
4. *Comparative need* is need which relates to equity between groups or individuals.

Twenty-six years on, a wide range of literature has been published around the concept (see Percy-Smith 1996). Bradshaw acknowledges the importance and relevance of all such critical debates, together with allied developments in perceptions and understanding. Doyal & Gough (1991), for example, explored the concept and suggested that need can be broken down into universal and intermediate aspects.

The universal needs relate to:

◆ Physical needs.
◆ Autonomy.

The intermediate needs relate to:

◆ Adequate nutritional food.
◆ Clean water.
◆ Non-hazardous physical environment.
◆ Appropriate health care.
◆ Security in childhood.
◆ Significant primary relationships.
◆ Physical activity.
◆ Economic security.
◆ Appropriate education.
◆ State birth control and child bearing.

Many other analysts also have attempted to create such lists of needs, and also to differentiate between needs, wants, interests and desires, (Townsend 1979, Sen 1981). What becomes quickly apparent is that there is a multitude of perceptions around the concept of need, and that these are influenced by personal beliefs or judgements on the relative importance of different needs, and the priority accorded to them as a result. In relation to health care allocation, resources   may well be distributed according to the particular emphasis pursued in the health need assessment.

Three models of assessing need include:

◆ A medical/epidemiological model.
◆ An economic model.
◆ A social model.

These models also implicitly reflect a perspective on the nature of health and health care as discussed in earlier chapters. We will look at each model in turn.

A MEDICAL/EPIDEMIOLOGICAL MODEL FOR NEEDS ASSESSMENT

In this model the focus is on the presence or absence of disease (Helman 1981, Long 1984). An individual will be considered to have needs if they are ill, and experience a desire to use available health care services. This model reflects a medical definition of health and of need, and responses allocated to any individual will relate to the provision of caring services and the curing of disease.

AN ECONOMIC MODEL FOR NEEDS ASSESSMENT

In this model the emphasis is on the effective and appropriate allocation of scarce financial resources to meet assessed need. It is based on an assumption that all assessed health need (using epidemiological surveys and methods) cannot be met because there will always be insufficient resources. The emphasis then is on prioritising the assessed levels of need in relation to some cost–benefit analysis, and in turn allocating services in the most economically effective way. The aim is to achieve maximum benefit for minimum cost. Ineffective or costly interventions are likely to be discontinued if their value is unproven, and rationing of services will be carried out by the use of economic indicators and values.

A SOCIAL MODEL FOR NEEDS ASSESSMENT

The perception of need which underpins this model is holistic in nature. It is based on an appreciation of the eclectic determinants of health and health need, and the ways is which these open up the scope for potential care interventions. It is focused on people's needs for health and well-being, and not just on services and diseases. Those who adhere to a social model of need highlight the importance of the lay person's own perceptions of need, rather than relying on the professional view or indeed that of the economic analyst. The response to need is very much concerned with the development of an individual's ability (or that of the community) to realise life's aspirations and ambitions. It looks to the creation of a supportive environment which will encourage such growth. Bradshaw (1994) explains the focus of this model well. He says:

> *Need is not an absolute state, not just an untreated condition, not just an impairment or a disability, but also an absence of well-being or quality of life. Meeting need is not the treatment of disease, but whether the quality of life is enhanced as a result. For the most efficient meeting of health needs, we may need to look beyond improvements in detection, diagnosis, care, medical delivery and even prevention and health education, to changes in the social structure itself – to changes in the material conditions in which people live and the life chances they have available to them. Self reports – the experience, assessments and subjective feelings of people (their felt needs) – have greater importance and validity.*

Brief reflections to all three models

The models then in different ways suggest how need is viewed, and in turn provide a focus or rationale for making allocative decisions on the health care resources available. The epidemiologists/economists, for example, would see the social model as much too ambitious and nebulous to be helpful or realistic in relation either to the appropriate distribution of resources, or in providing some boundaries of responsibility for NHS care.

In turn, supporters of the social model would refer to the limited perspectives of the other two frameworks. On the one hand, they say the epidemiological/medical model sees needs in a unidimensional way, and focuses on disease, secondary and tertiary interventions and health services. On the other hand, the economists use this limited epidemiological perspective and then further coldly define, weigh and prioritise need in relation to the available scarce financial resources for health and health care. According to Foreman (1996):

> *The economic model effectively replaces needs with the more restricted concept of priorities. This . . . throws up difficult questions about how priorities should be set and who should have access to health care.*

During the period of reform the previous Government used a combination of the epidemiological and economic models, with some aspects taken from

the social approach. Foreman (1986) described this 'hybrid model' as empha-
sising the role of existing services and the views of experts, resulting in a
limited understanding of need, and in turn, confining potential change to
the modification of existing services. This view, of course, reflects the previously stated assertion that the parameters of NHS care have been further constrained and often reduced by the impact of government health and
economic policy reforms – in spite of many assertions to the contrary.

On this final point, we now turn to look at the historical usage and interpretation of need in the allocation of health care resources. Hopefully, this
will help to aid consideration of the application of the theoretical concept in
real life situations in the NHS over time.

THE HISTORICAL USAGE OF THE CONCEPT OF NEED IN HEALTH CARE DELIVERY

*I think it is appropriate to remember what health care choices were really
like before the National Health Service, and that the NHS was put here to
stand in place in fear. (Clay 1988)*

The late Trevor Clay (General Secretary RCN) published an article just over
a decade ago, in celebration of the 40th anniversary of the creation of the
National Health Service (NHS) on 5 July 1948. He reminded his nurse read-
ership of its many obvious achievements since that time, and not least that
the fear of the costs of ill health did not now hang over the lives and everyday actions of people today, as it often did in pre-NHS times. He pondered
ruefully on the fact that a generation of people under 50 had no memory or
clear understanding of the hardship and dilemmas faced by many, when they
or their families had health needs which could not be met. Reasons for this
included:

◆ An inability to raise the money to pay for medical care.
◆ A lack of local, appropriate or affordable services.

Health needs for many often went unmet, particularly among the least well
off, with morbidity and mortality rates reflecting the seriousness of the situation all too clearly. In 1941, Huxley described in the 'Picture Post' how life was
overwhelmingly difficult for many of the poorest mothers in Britain at that
time. He noted:

*An appallingly large number of working class mothers persist in carrying
on when they are not really fit, because they feel that, for the sake of their
man and their children, they cannot afford not to carry on. Careful surveys
have shown that nearly half of such women are in a state of definitely bad*

health, and only about a quarter really well. It is only by removing such fears and frustrations that we can hope to reduce the alarming spread of neurosis and mental ill-health in general. (Huxley 1941)

The Beveridge Report published in 1942, a year after Huxley's article, provided an introduction to the proposed creation of welfare structures in response to the health related needs which faced many of the British public. Beveridge referred collectively to these needs as the 'Five Giants': Want, Ignorance, Disease, Idleness and Squalor (Beveridge 1942). The post-war Labour Government's policy response to these needs thus involved the creation of a benefits system, improved schools for all, employment and job creation, a housing plan for new buildings and, of course, a national health service.

Overall, it is fair to conclude that the 1945–51 Government's response to the perceived needs of the population was, in part, the creation of a wide-ranging public health agenda covering all the major determinants of health need. The concept of need as applied then was thus a broad social model, reflecting a belief that people needed to be helped to health, and to help each other in turn, in many different ways. The values which underpinned the welfare reforms exemplified an acknowledgement of, and general responsibility for, each member of society, collectively insuring against the personal, financial and social costs of the unexpected, ill health and other misfortune. They said the meeting of individual needs through the welfare system involved notions of responsibilities as well as rights. As Beveridge (1942) had explained:

The plan is not one for giving to everybody something for nothing, or will free recipients from personal responsibilities. It leaves room and encouragement to all individuals to win something above the national minimum, to find out and to satisfy new and higher needs than bare physical needs.

The identification and meeting of socially defined need was thus the raison d'être for the welfare state, and a rationale for the allocation of publicly financed welfare services, including health care. While then, health care services were to be free at the point of need, they were not free, but paid for by taxation. At this point it is worth remembering that there was political, professional and public opposition to the Labour Government's collective response to need in the form of the Welfare State. It can be argued that although the political opposition was defeated in the 1940s, making way for a new consensus which lasted until the 1970s, the individualist response in the 1980s to the perceived problems of the Welfare State repeated many of the earlier arguments of the 1940s.

Initially then the assessment of levels of health need was determined by health professional and researcher alike. At this stage their interpretations provided adequate evidence on which to base government decisions on the allocation of health care resources, and there was some degree of political consensus for this approach. It was assumed that once individuals had accessed the new health service and received appropriate attention, then their demands would reduce, and costs would fall. As such, according to O'Keefe, Ottewill & Wall (1994) government interest in the NHS revolved around NHS finance and organisational matters. As time moved on, however, concerns around the ever increasing public demand for health care services began to influence and to focus government thinking, not least on the cost of keeping its promised responsibility for meeting all health needs. While politically it was important to maintain the concept of need as a guiding rationale for the NHS, the cost of meeting assessed needs was becoming too high a price to sustain, for whichever government was in power.

The growing concerns around the funding of the health service, and indeed other public sector bodies, should be set against the backcloth of the development of a general economic crisis during the late 1960s and early 1970s. The cross-party political consensus in support of the NHS lasted until this period. However, the apparent underperformance of the economy was seen by the political right as resulting from high public sector spending and direct taxation (Fatchett 1994). This situation provided right wing politicians with the opportunity to reassess their agendas and priorities in relation to all public spending areas, including the NHS. They argued that if NHS activity remained uncontrolled, then it would consume ever-increasing amounts of public sector monies, to the detriment of other important welfare programmes. In addition, while then the popular focus on meeting need would continue in principle in the NHS, the interpretation and application of the concept was perceived as needing some redefinition and organisational planning.

During the 1970s formal planning structures were introduced to take control of the health service which appeared to be facing unlimited demands, and seemingly spinning down a black hole of ever-increasing expenditure. O'Keefe, Ottewill & Wall (1994) reminds us of a number of initiatives which effectively began to redefine, to quantify, to constrain and to determine the parameters of need for which the NHS was to be responsible in the subsequent years. The initiatives created were:

◆ Preparation of long-term plans by local authorities for health and welfare services.
◆ Establishment of NHS planning systems.
◆ Introduction of joint planning initiatives.
◆ Setting of objectives in relation to needs:
  – health and social care priorities (Department of Health and Social Security 1976a);

- children and young people (Department of Health and Social Security 1976b);
- health education and promotion (Department of Health and Social Security 1976c).

THE 1980S AND 1990S: THE REFORMS AND A NEW PERSPECTIVE ON NEED

During the 1980s and 1990s, the planning of NHS activity has become increasingly financially driven in relation to meeting need. The pursuit of cost efficiency, effectiveness and value for money has become the influential and guiding motive. That said, while according to many the founding principles of the NHS have been compromised in this pursuit of economic goals, all four Conservative governments continued to state their continuing commitment and adherence to the values of the NHS, not least to meeting the needs of clients free at the point of need (Cmd 3425 1996).

The implementation of health service reforms, including both management (Griffiths 1983) and the creation of the internal health care market (Cmd 555 1989), has provided the opportunity to redefine the nature of the organisation, to strengthen the power of management and government, and to set out the parameters of need that professionals should be expected to address. The changes have encouraged a questioning of patterns of delivery and resource allocation, and the effectiveness of services provided. The assessment of need also was found to be wanting. Need as a guiding concept was to be measured in a more systematic and scientific way, and to move away from the qualitative nature of previous interpretations. Specific guidance on assessing need was provided by the NHSME (1991). Foreman (1996) described the technique proposed as 'hybrid'. She said:

> It is based primarily on the traditional epidemiological method, but is strongly influenced by economic approaches and some aspects of the social model.

As she also stated:

> The aim is to assess not only the needs of the population, but also the cost effectiveness of the services provided. Thus the epidemiological and economic approaches are combined in an attempt to encourage the provision of services which most cost effectively maximise the health of the population.

It would seem that the whole thrust of the Conservative health reforms has been about redefining the concept of need, not least into a slimmer version than in previous times. It is worth mentioning, for example, three important health documents which have helped to set out the concept in line with accepted government thinking. The documents were:

1. 'The Health of the Nation' (Cmd 1986 1992).
2. 'The Patient's Charter' (Department of Health 1991).
3. 'Local Voices' (NHSME 1992).

The first two, discussed in other chapters, provided several important themes. In 'The Health of the Nation' (Cmd 1986 1992), for example, the government presented its broad definition of health, in line with that of the World Health Organization (WHO 1985). At the same time it clarified the specific role and contribution of the NHS in achieving that very wide ranging social goal. The NHS and the Government could not, and would not, be responsible for all health needs in the population.

As Bottomley put it:

Although there is much that the Government and the NHS need to do, the objectives and targets cannot be delivered by Government and the NHS alone. They are truly for the nation, for all of us to achieve. We must be clear about where responsibilities lie. We must get the balance right between what the Government, and Government alone, can do, what other organisations and agencies need to do, and finally, what individuals and families themselves must contribute if the strategy is to succeed. (Cmd 1986 1992)

The NHS was expected to play its part in 'working for patients', and to contribute wherever possible to other extra-NHS health-focused collaborative ventures with wider contributor organisations and the general public.

In a similarly defining approach, the Government framed the expected nature of the NHS contribution in meeting consumer need by publishing 'The Patient's Charter' (Department of Health 1991). The proposed aim was to ensure that each consumer had the power to insist that their health needs were met appropriately and to a high standard. In turn, advice was given to the then existing district health authorities (DHAs) and family health service authorities (FHSAs) on how to make the services responsive to the needs, views and preferences of the people in their localities. The document, 'Local Voices' (NHSME 1992) provided ideas on how greater involvement by local people could be achieved, and their voices brought into the debates on meeting need. As the document stated:

If health authorities are to establish a champion of the people role, their decisions should reflect, as far as practical, what people want, their preferences, concerns and values. Being responsive to local views will enhance the credibility of health authorities, but more importantly, is likely to result in services which are better suited to local needs and are therefore more appropriate.

So did this happen?

We will now consider the veracity of claims to an increasingly needs led service during the period of NHS reform up to April 1997.

THE REFORMS: NEEDS LED? OR MARKET LED?

During the whole period up to April 1997 few nurses in practice will have been unaware of the apparently opposing objectives of Conservative health care policy. The assessment and meeting of client need have not been immune from such distractions and dilemmas. On the one hand, care delivered was to be research proven, cost efficient and effective, quality laden, and to provide value for money. On the other hand, the purchase of care services from providers was to be based on an assessment of client needs and to be consumer led. While these objectives may seem reasonable, experience during the period of Conservative reform suggested a degree of incompatibility. Efforts made to introduce a more planned, quantifiable and commercialised corporate health care environment, sit uneasily with the notion of researching, assessing, planning, purchasing and delivering care based on the very 'contested and controversial' concept of need. After all, the control of public expenditure had been high on the agenda of successive Conservative governments. As such, it is difficult to see why any activity should have been pursued which was likely to increase expenditure, – and not least, that of responding to such an elastic concept as health need. The pursuit of any serious assessment of health need would surely create greater demands and expectations, which would add to, rather than detract from, the NHS bill. As Ottewill & Wall (1991) explain:

> *There are considerable resource implications in seeking to meet unexpressed needs, as well as responding to the demands from the public for treatment.*

They describe the process of assessing need as: 'A task almost without limit in terms of both scale and conceptual complexity'.

Explanations then for the apparent support for the difficult and potentially costly exercise of responding to the users' perceptions of need are worth some consideration. To start with, and on a positive note, some will feel that the dual objectives were perfectly reasonable. They reflected a balanced and sound approach to the assessment of need and to the delivery of appropriate and relevant health care. The application of value for money criteria would ensure that maximum benefit was gained for minimum cost. This reflects good management of public sector resources, and as such would help promote and maintain effective care services for everyone in need.

Another less positive interpretation of the stated objectives might be that the pursuit of the previous Government's economic goals for health care delivery, i.e. value for money and retrenchment in public sector spending, were in reality of greater importance in the health care equation than that of meeting health needs as defined by the general public. Many in practice may have felt that the pursuit of proven value for money initiatives, and adherence to budget by cost-conscious managers, have ensured that some of the more difficult to research and measure activity around user need has been sidelined in favour of the more easily measurable. As a result, some will have reached the unsurprising conclusion that the emphasis and importance given to the assessment of need exercise was merely a smoke-screen to cover up the more important objectives of cost containment, and the deliberate reduction in size of what would become more clearly defined as relevant activity in the business of the health service. That said, the previous Government could (and did) legitimately argue that the NHS focus on meeting need continued to be maintained, albeit in a more limited way than many practitioners and indeed the public may have liked. As North & Bradshaw (1997) remind us:

> *The concept of need possesses chameleon characteristics which enabled it to be adapted and moulded to the requirements of the market.*

As we now look forward to a new decade of reform as set out in the 1997 White Paper (Cmd 3807 1997), will the concept of health need be redefined again? Indeed, to use North's words, 'will the concept of need be "remoulded" to the requirements of the Government's new NHS?'

Where do we go from here?

It has been argued already that during the long period of Conservative health reform the concept of need which underpins NHS activity has been both redefined and reduced. The language of priority setting, efficiency and effectiveness, marketisation and the pursuit of value for money, has effectively redirected and reduced professional nurse care activity not least in response to assessed need. There has been a clear shift away from former more broadly based social and public health concerns, to an increasingly medically defined and limited illness business. While increased user involvement in decision making and needs assessment, together with consumer empowerment, have both been highlighted throughout the reforms, the reality has been very different. The economically driven agenda has created a financially tight context for care. The impact of this has been to reduce rather than expand client choice, and in turn has redefined the concept of need and thus the business of the NHS in a more limited way than hitherto.

THE FUTURE: 'THE NEW NHS. MODERN, DEPENDABLE' (CMD 3807 1997)

The White Paper 'The New NHS' was published late in 1997. It set out the Government's plans for health services for the next decade, and like all of its predecessors was both supportive and full of promise. As the Prime Minister put it:

> *As we approach the fiftieth anniversary of the NHS, it is time to reflect on the huge achievements of the NHS. But in a changing world no organisation, however great, can stand still. The NHS needs to modernise in order to meet the demands of today's public. This White Paper begins a process of modernisation. The NHS will start to provide new and better services to the public.*

Very specifically then for this discussion, the proposed 10-year programme seems to offer a different perception and emphasis on the concept of need – one which appears broader than has been offered by all governments in the recent past. For example, in the opening statement (1.1), it is made clear that the NHS will be concerned directly with both health and illness, and in reducing health inequalities. This is a major change of focus for the NHS in relation to meeting need, one which reflects strongly the social model of health need assessment as discussed earlier. The document states quite clearly that the new service will be:

> *A national health service which offers people high quality treatment and care when they need it. An NHS that does not just treat people when they are ill, but works with others to improve health and reduce inequalities.*

It has to be said that this statement is very different from those made by Bottomley in 'The Health of the Nation' (Cmd 1986 1992), in which she appeared to define the responsibility of the NHS in meeting need in a much more limited and illness-focused way. By contrast, the Government demonstrates throughout the White Paper its intention to create a broader, less competitive, more collaborative, health-focused agenda, one which responds to issues of health need which are much wider than illness and hospital services. This view is reinforced in Section 1:2.

> *Achieving this vision means we have to change our approach to tackling ill-health and inequality. The Government will ensure the NHS works locally with those who provide social care, housing, education and employment; just as the Government itself will work nationally across Whitehall to bring about lasting improvements in the public's health.*

In the White Paper the Government stated on many occasions (as have previous governments, of course) that the needs of patients will be central to the new NHS. That said, a major change might be able to be introduced in order to achieve this goal. This involves the replacement of the internal health care market, its economic imperatives and ideological values, by a system of integrated care. This new approach, it is suggested, will not only reduce the overheavy bureaucracy of administering the competitive relationships of trusts, but focus activity on meeting the needs of clients rather than on accountancy issues and balancing budgets.

It is also proposed that the voice and views on needs as expressed by the public will be harnessed more strongly than ever before. There is a repeated emphasis on public and health professional partnerships in care. The Government wants:

> *A strong public voice in health and health care decision-making, recognising the important part played by Community Health Councils in providing information and advice, and in representing the patient's interests.*

The restated support for the Community Health Council, who since 1974 have represented the interests of the public, is another important sign of the Government's wish to respond to user need in the future development of the NHS. Further, they intend to secure informed public and expert involvement in planning local services. Rather than relying on economic indicator or professional decision, the aim will be to provide the opportunity for the general public to define local need, and to be part of the decision making and implementation of policy at local levels. The development of health action zones, primary care groups and health improvement programmes all provide and require room for the involvement of the public. Indeed, the creation of this type of open environment in relation to all NHS bodies and their working, appears qualitatively different from the secretive atmosphere of trusts and health authority boardrooms in the past 8 years.

DRAWING TOGETHER THE STRANDS

At the beginning of this discussion it was argued that the concept of need (albeit difficult to define either precisely or to everyone's satisfaction) should provide a focus for health care delivery, which embodies a broad perspective on the determinants of health need. The creation of the NHS as one part of the welfare state was perceived as a demonstration of that vision.

That said, the old and well-established pre-NHS health care roots ensured that responses to the health of the population were to be fundamentally medically defined and illness focused. This legacy shaped and coloured responses to health need until the late 1970s. From that point onward, the planning of NHS activity became increasingly financially driven. The pursuit of cost efficiency, effectiveness and value for money became influential and guiding motives. The impact of this, it was argued, was to reduce rather than to expand responses to the needs of clients.

By contrast, the present Government's perception of the concept of need, and thus its response to it, is being moulded into a shape which is different from that of recent years. The thrust taken by the previous governments, not least with its strong emphasis on the economic and epidemiological frameworks for need and care, does in retrospect look very narrow as compared with the new proposed way forward – that of the social model. The changes proposed will not be easy to carry through, not least because of the enormity and the complexity of the task proposed. The Government itself acknowledges this fact:

> *This is a tough and challenging programme. On some fronts there will be early progress. Others may be for a long haul. Some may take time to show visible improvement. But the end result will be an NHS that responds to a changed and changing world. Where patients can expect services to be quickly available of consistently high quality. Where medical advance can be harnessed and made more locally available. When care is there for people when they need it.*

Defining need in turn defines the parameters of any health service. If successive governments have tended to lean upon narrower definitions of health, this might be inevitable, given the constant constraints upon public spending. A wider definition of need may achieve both public spending savings in the long term, and improved satisfaction of health care service users. To achieve this ideal, as promised by the current Government, will require a significant short-term financial and political investment. Change is therefore not going to be easy. If, however, it is achieved, the wider definition of need will necessarily influence beneficially the role definition of nurses, their education and training. The social model of need, to which reference has been made in this chapter, and to which the current government presently seems committed, will open for nurses a positive interaction between their own role, and others operating in other social structures, such as employment, education and housing.

REFERENCES

Bevan A 1952 In place of fear. Heinemann, London
Beveridge W 1942 The Beveridge report on social insurance. 1 December. HMSO, London
Bradshaw J 1972 The concept of social need. New Society. 30 March, pp 640–643
Bradshaw J 1994 The conceptualisation and measurement of need. A social policy perspective. In: Poppay J, Williams G (eds) Researching people's health. Routledge, London
Clay T 1988 Freedom from fear. Nursing Times 84(27): 19
Command 555 1989 Working for Patients. Department of Health, London
Command 1986 1992 The Health of the Nation: a strategy for health in England. Department of Health, London

Command 3425 1996 The National Health Service: a service with ambitions. Department of Health, London

Command 3807 1997 The New NHS: Modern. Dependable. Department of Health, London

Department of Health 1991 The Patient's Charter. HMSO, London

Department of Health and Social Security 1976a Priorities for health and personal social services in England. HMSO, London

Department of Health and Social Security 1976b Fit for the future: the report of the committee on child health services. HMSO, London

Department of Health and Social Security 1976c Prevention and health. Everybody's business. A reassessment of public and personal health. HMSO, London

Doyal L, Gough I 1991 A theory of human need. Macmillan, London

Fatchett A 1994 Politics, policy and nursing. Baillière Tindall, London

Foreman Anne 1996 In: Percy-Smith J (ed) Needs assessment in public policy. Open University, Milton Keynes, ch 5, p 66

Griffiths R 1983 The NHS management inquiry. DHSS, London

Helman CG 1981 Disease versus illness in general practice. Journal of Royal College of General Practitioners 31: 548

Huxley 1941 Picture Post 10(1): 4 January

Long A 1984 Research into health and illness. Gower, London

Maslow A 1954 Motivation and personality. Harper Row, New York

NHSME National Health Service Management Executive 1991 Assessing health care needs. DoH, London

NHSME National Health Service Management Executive 1992 Local voices. The views of local people in purchasing for health. DoH, London

North N, Bradshaw Y 1997 Perspectives in health care. Macmillan, Basingstoke

O'Keefe E, Ottewill R, Wall A 1994 Community health: issues in management. Business Education Publishers, Sunderland, Tyne and Wear

Ottewill R, Wall A 1991 The growth and development of community health services. Business Education Publishers, Sunderland, Tyne and Wear

Percy-Smith J (ed) 1996 Needs assessment in public policy. Open University Press, Milton Keynes

Sanderson I 1996 In: Percy-Smith (ed) Needs assessment in public policy. Open University, Milton Keynes, pp 11–31

Sen A K 1981 Food and famine: a essay on entitlement and deprivation. Oxford University Press, London

Townsend P 1979 Poverty in the United Kingdom. Penguin, Harmondsworth

United Kingdom Central Council 1992 Code of professional conduct for the nurse, midwife and health visitor. UKCC, London

WHO 1985 Targets for health for all. WHO, Copenhagen

5

Consumer empowerment

The stated purpose of the National Health Service (NHS) reforms of the 1980s and the 1990s was to provide the users of the service with better quality health care and a wider choice of services. It was clearly set out in the then Prime Minister's foreword to the White Paper 'Working for Patients' (Cmd 555 1989) that all the proposals were designed to put the needs of the patients first. This was a continuation of the often previously stated desire to strengthen the users' position through the provision of increased information, and the development of a more commercialised approach in health care delivery. This is evident, for example, both through the introduction of general management principles following the NHS Management Inquiry (Griffiths 1983) and the subsequent development of family practitioner services as set out in the 1987 White Paper, 'Promoting Better Health' (Cmd 249 1987).

As we now approach the millennium, notions of consumerism and empowerment are popular concepts that continue to permeate the health care agenda. Having acknowledged this, it is worthwhile to ponder on the difficulty of defining in absolute terms either of these concepts, and in turn making them a reality in practice. It would seem that politicians, policy makers, health care professionals, managers and the general public alike have latched onto specific aspects which reflect their understanding (or which best suit their purpose) of the concepts of consumerism or empowerment within the health care setting. Whether or not the users of the health services have in fact become active consumers or have been further empowered as a result of the reforms, depends greatly on subjective assessment. There is substantial scope for debate. While some believe that the creation of the internal health care market has resulted in much increased consumer power, others refer to the creation of an illusion of power, to the supermarket model of consumerism (Winkler 1987), to the frills and trappings of patient power (Fatchett 1994).

Today the arguments continue unabated. Because of this, some initial comment must be made about the nature of the concept of consumerism, and not least its appropriateness and applicability to health care delivery. The first part of the discussion to follow will be entitled: 'Consumerism and health care: compatible concepts?' This will lead into a number of discussions which will examine the thesis of enhanced consumer choice within the health services. The headings for the broad areas to be covered include the following:

1. Why examine the concept in practice?
2. Policy developments leading up to the NHS reforms of the 1990s:
   - creation to denigration: 1948–79
   - the General Election of 1979
   - the introduction of general management: 1984
   - the creation of the internal health care market: 1989 and onwards.
3. The consumers and the reforms: efforts to empower.
4. A judgement so far.
5. The 1997 General Election: courting the electorate.
6. 'The new NHS. Modern, Dependable' (Cmd 3807 1997).
7. An agenda for nurses: the challenge for the future.

As we consider the evidence and the arguments, we may be led to conclude that the system created as a result of the changes within the NHS has not necessarily empowered either consumer or professional nurse. We may also conclude that in any case, a distributive system which is based upon a vicarious relationship between individuals and providers cannot in itself be guaranteed to add to consumer power and choice. Finally, and against this background, we will look at the consumer empowerment argument, and to the changes which have taken place, and how these relate to the experience and role of professional nurses, not least in their quest to empower both the clients, and indeed themselves, during the period of Conservative health care reform.

CONSUMERISM AND HEALTH CARE: COMPATIBLE CONCEPTS?

First, we need to question the basic assumption that health and health care are like any other commodity to be bought and sold in the marketplace. Every individual is seen as a powerful consumer, because he has money to spend on the services on offer. Linked to this is the notion that the potential user of health services can, or should, be expected to play the role of active consumer, and in effect, 'go shopping' to buy health care as and when the need arises. Unsurprisingly, many have strongly criticised the use of the term 'consumer' in the context of health care delivery (Klein 1980, Winkler 1987, Normand 1991, Fatchett 1994). Abel-Smith (1976), for example, in his analysis concluded:

> *There are few fields of consumer expenditure where the consumer is as ill-equipped to exercise this theoretical sovereignty as in the health services.*

So, what 'equipment' might be needed by a true consumer in a free market model of health care? Consumer needs could be summarised as:

◆ Adequate information.
◆ A practical range of alternative services and interventions.
◆ The ability to make a rational choice.
◆ The opportunity to select from a variety of options.
◆ The ability to compare the quality of one service or intervention with another.
◆ Legal protection.
◆ The ability to have a refund.
◆ The ability to take action to seek redress or compensation, if product, treatment or intervention failed to work, was inappropriate, or did not reach the quality standard promised and expected.

While it is easy to see how some of these would be relevant, appropriate and possible for many individuals – perhaps the fittest, the most articulate, and the financially solvent, however – there are still problems worthy of consideration. As Normand states:

> *Where health is bought and sold as a commodity, it fails on several counts – and not least, if one believes in the principle that care should be given to those in need, and that some equitable approach should apply in its delivery (see United Kingdom Central Council 1992).*

It would appear that the free market is also seen as poor at allocating resources to those most in need of health care. Having said that, others would argue that the same applies to the centrally controlled distribution of NHS resources. Research has demonstrated time after time that the inverse care law and health inequality continue sadly to apply (Black 1980, Benzeval, Judge & Whitehead 1996, Dorling 1997). In this situation, those who need the most help to be healthy, the poorest in society, appear to gain the least from the health care resources made available in any particular society, whatever the method of distribution. The more well off and articulate, by contrast, are more able to access any health promoting structures available, and in turn to achieve a better health status than those who lack such attributes and opportunities.

Linked to all of the above, is the issue of illness and poor health being correlated with low socioeconomic status and poverty. Those who suffer ill health and fall into this category, may be unable to afford to buy much needed services, albeit available in the market. To compound this issue still further, the commercial judgement of those who insure against the cost of ill health, and who fund private health care, may be to charge such groups higher premiums than low risk groups, or even to refuse them insurance cover because of the possibility of them developing very costly illnesses in the long term, for example, people with HIV.

Another important point to consider is that a free market cannot, and does not, aspire to meet the overarching and general health needs of a whole community, rich and poor alike. There is a tendency to offer care to meet specific health needs only, and to provide these services within areas of appropriate consumer prosperity. Poorer areas of population are less likely to offer commercially attractive sites, or indeed sources of potential income. Because of this, many consumers, and probably the poorest, may have little or no choice of health care provision, either because it does not exist in their own area, or because of an inability to pay for services elsewhere. While this situation may be satisfactory in relation to buying biscuits or designer clothes, in health care this may mean the difference between a long life or an early death depending on the financial and social situation. As such, many would argue that health care is a different and special good or commodity, and that it should therefore be allocated on the basis of need, rather than on the ability to pay. The creation of the NHS in 1948 was a prime example of such a view.

It is also worth considering the belief that the individual consumer of health care in a free market is ipso facto more powerful than a patient/client in a publicly funded and centrally directed setting. This may be a misplaced belief. All individuals, whatever the health care setting, lack information and expertise in health matters. It is the professional providers of care who have the monopoly of knowledge and skills, or why would anyone pay for their attention? Health professionals clearly have greater power because of their special understanding, and, if this is abused for commercial gain, for example, it can and does lead to an exploitation of the consumers or an oversupply of care services.

In conclusion, the free market may theoretically offer the opportunity, finance permitting, for any individual consumer to be treated when, where and how they would like. However, the patient will be reliant upon the provider to determine the degree, type and quality of care deemed appropriate and necessary. The theoretical idea of the active consumer being the more powerful player in the client–provider relationship is open to debate, and will surely depend on an individual's ability and knowledge and financial resources. For the majority of the population seeking health care, the power relationship will be weighted in favour of the provider who has the experience being sought. This will apply whether in the private market or in the public sector. It begins to become apparent, then, that both sectors may have interests which overlap.

Potter (1988) has proposed that a number of convenient principles implicit within a free market could be readily applied to a centrally directed health sector such as the NHS. These include issues around:

◆ Access.
◆ Choice.
◆ Information.
◆ Redress.
◆ Participation.

The interpretation and appreciation of these in practice will reflect the philosophy or ideology underpinning the policy and legislative programmes of any particular government. What is clear, however, is that different governments may create differing policy responses to apparently the same problems. Policy activity is not value free, but reflects a particular ideological perspective. As the Labour Government's collectivist policy responses to the health problems and needs of the 1940s reflected their political views and judgement, so the Conservative Governments of the 1980s and 1990s have reformed the NHS, and on their terms, empowered the consumers. They have worked openly to minimise public sector involvement in health care, to release the energies and competition of a free market environment. At the same time they have aimed to maximise personal/individual responsibilities for health and health care, thus empowering the consumer. Whether this has been achieved is still very much open to debate.

WHY EXAMINE THE CONCEPT IN PRACTICE?

A discussion of the apparently new style consumer responsiveness implied by the NHS changes is worthwhile and relevant both for nurses and other NHS employees. As we are all aware, for nearly two decades NHS reform has been underpinned by the emphasis on an apparently newly found belief in the importance of the wishes of the individual consumer of health care. This reflects a faith in each person's ability to choose between competing health service options, and their power to force the providers of health care to be responsive to their expressed needs. The veracity of the outcome of these claims needs to be examined. In reality has it happened at all like this?

Indeed, have the reforms within the NHS and, in turn, the nursing profession offered anything new and empowering to clients? After all, putting the patient first, it is claimed, has always been central to nurse caring. The current code of conduct (United Kingdom Central Council 1992) reaffirmed clearly that the primacy of the interests of patients or clients remains quite properly the dominant theme (Pyne 1992). Without a doubt, other professionals would surely defend their own long term position *vis-à-vis* their clients in a similar vein.

However, defensive protestations by professionals that they have always put their clients first, and that the reforms have made no positive difference to their approach to the users of services, are perhaps at the worst indiscreet and foolish, and at the best, hopefully, telling an untruth. It is worth remembering that prior to the start of the reform process, the NHS was not seen as user responsive and fault free. Many analysts acknowledge the lack of user voice and power in both organisational development and delivery of service. North & Bradshaw (1997) referred to 'the bleak habitat of the would-be consumer', and Klein (1989) to the 'ghosts in the NHS machinery.' Professional groups, doctors, nurses, and allied professionals, decided who received what, how and when, and the users had little influence or say (Pollitt 1989). This was a point reiterated by the Griffiths Management Inquiry Team (Griffiths 1983). The so-called 'users voice' in the form of community health councils created in 1974 have also had little power. Indeed, they have been described as 'toothless watchdogs', and merely 'throwers of grit into the machinery of the NHS.' (Klein 1989). While the promise of consumer centrality has been made by many on many occasions during the recent past, it seems that claims and practice have not gone hand in hand. It is evident that there is still much work to do, as Donaldson (1995) reminds us:

> *There is a long way to go before what the public wants, and what the health service provides are better matched.*

If that is the case, then the discussion to follow is of relevance to all nurses who, like Pyne, seek to uphold their code of conduct, and to reaffirm in a serious and meaningful way the primacy of the interests of patients/clients. For, unless we consider the attributes, characteristics, uses and abuses of consumer empowerment both within the NHS, and within professional practice, then any desire for truly effective client empowerment is unlikely to be achieved in the foreseeable future.

We now turn to a discussion of the policy developments leading up to and around the reforms within the NHS in which the concept of consumer power was very much on the agenda.

POLICY DEVELOPMENTS LEADING UP TO THE NHS REFORMS OF THE 1990s

Creation to denigration: 1948–79

British governments of all political persuasions accepted and indeed promoted without hesitation and question the development of the NHS up until the early 1980s. However, from this point onward, the developing backcloth of concern about rising government expenditure and criticism of the scale and scope of all arms of the welfare state, and government intervention in general, began to impact upon the NHS. It became a target for both cost-containment programmes and organisational reform. This reflected a desire to control expenditure on health which was seen to be high and rising, with demographic trends promising a massive growth in health care spending on a proportionately growing elderly population. In addition, technological development and innovation with an ever-continuing growth in the range of life-enhancing and extending treatments potentially on offer within the NHS, threatened also to push the cost of NHS care out of control. Concerns about such issues only served to validate the growing view held by those on the political right, that the NHS specifically and the welfare state in general provided a damning combination of all those negative aspects which were contributing to Britain's continuing economic decline. The cost and the nature of state welfare were seen as putting a dead hand on the financial entrepreneurialism of Britain's market potential, both in the national and international field.

Sheldon (1980) in his work set out a picture of the NHS which, without a doubt, reflected the beliefs about it held by many in the Conservative Party. It was seen to be bureaucratic, unresponsive, inert, resisting of change, with appalling industrial relations, and it was perceived as not encouraging of any individual sense of responsibility for health.

Butler (1992) in his analysis refers to:

◆ The heavy influence of central and local bureaucracies.
◆ The restrictive practices of powerful professions.
◆ The indifference to the quality of care and services provided.
◆ The lack of incentives for innovation and efficiency.
◆ The deadening reliance upon government funds.

Finally, and importantly for this particular discussion, he refers also to the absence of real consumer choice.

Alongside the critical academic debate, right wing politicians and much of the tabloid press during the early 1980s offered an often derogatory liturgy of accusation against the NHS and the other arms of the welfare state. They were described as wasteful organisations which swallowed up hard-earned amounts of taxpayers' money. They were accused of providing inappropriate and wasteful services, and financial help to people who could, if they really tried, look after themselves and their families instead of relying upon the so-called 'Nanny State.' These sorts of views were widely promoted and for many in the population held great appeal. Debates on public spending and all the attendant ills during and after the 1979 election period found a receptive audience in the population at large. The NHS was not immune. As Sheldon (1980) concluded:

> *It (the NHS) does not supply the British people with the best medical care they want, because it prevents them as individual consumers from paying for the services that suit their personal circumstances, requirements and preferences.*

The General Election of 1979

The Conservative Party's 1979 election promises of reduced public spending, decreased direct taxation, and thus more choice and freedom for individuals to spend their incomes as they wished, were clear signs to a new direction in health and spending policy. It was obvious that many of the electorate liked the messages which they heard, and returned a Conservative Government to power with a comfortable majority in the House of Commons. They were given a strong mandate for, among many other things, the creation of a different approach to health care organisation and delivery which, as we now know, was to have profound implications for the NHS, for all health professionals including nurses, and, by definition, for all consumers of health services. Few nurses will be unaware of the changes since then, with the creation of new structures, a different style of management coupled with the language of the marketplace, and the stated purpose to please the consumer.

Changing the NHS

The new Conservative Government was fully aware of the politically sensitive nature of changing the NHS. Its continuing popularity as a national institution made wholesale privatisation, for example, politically impossible (see North & Bradshaw 1997). However, while providing reassurance as to its safety and integrity, the Government started on changes which would be necessary for the creation of a new style business-like health service. They looked to develop it into an organisation which they believed would be better equipped to deal with the complex health issues and agendas of the 1980s and 1990s – not least, one which would be responsive to the interests of both taxpayer and health care consumer alike. The introduction of general management and all its attendant attributes was felt to be a major step in the right direction.

The introduction of general management: 1984

The introduction of general management as already discussed in an earlier chapter was a necessary first part of NHS change, a prerequisite for new developments to follow, subsequent to the NHS review of 1988. The Government believed that in order to run a consumer responsive health service, managers with business acumen were needed at every level to make it happen. Indeed the Inquiry Team had concluded that the NHS suffered from 'institutional stagnation.' While it was felt that business people had a keen sense of how well they were looking after their customers, it doubted that NHS management even tried to meet the needs of either patients or the community they served. The NHS, it believed, was not consumer friendly. There was a lack of information about services available, little choice of care on offer, no easily identified channels for complaints, and little effort made to find out about or to involve the recipients of the service. The Inquiry Team's solution to the problems created by this lack of consumer care was, as we know, the introduction of general management and a more business-like approach. Allsop (1996) described the general manager's task in detail:

> to provide a driving force for developing management plans, taking personal responsibility for providing appropriate levels of service; ensuring the quality of care; meeting budgets; achieving cost improvements; increasing productivity; monitoring performance and rewarding staff; ensuring research and development; and initiating measures to assess health outputs.

The aim of the task was that the consumer become central to all activities, and taxpayers gained best value for money.

What was needed

The Griffiths team believed that the consumers needed to be the central focus of health care delivery, and as such should be informed, consulted and encouraged to participate in all decision making – in fact, to become active consumers of health care, rather than the passive health service recipients they had become over time. As in the private sector, in business and industry, managers would need to seek the views of the consumers by means of market research, user surveys, meetings to give and receive information, lifestyle questionnaires, and other research projects. Interestingly, the Inquiry Team was dismissive of, and unimpressed by, the activity of the community health councils (CHCs). These had been created during the 1974 reorganisation of the NHS to increase democracy in the NHS through the 'representation of interests' of the users of the NHS (Allsop 1996). With few resources and little power however, many commentators had found their contribution limited (Shultz & Harrison 1983). The Inquiry Team saw the CHSs as 'labyrinthine and often unproductive.'

The Government's response to Griffiths

The rapid acceptance of the Inquiry Team's analysis of the failures of the NHS, and in turn its prospects for the introduction of a general managerial style and processes usually found in the private sector, was of no great surprise. The Government's right wing philosophy which underpinned all of its policy making, especially in relation to the public sector, ensured an appreciative audience for the Griffiths team's findings. While no doubt wholesale privatisation would have had even greater appeal to many in the wider Conservative Party, the Government took the lesser but equally important route opened up by the Griffiths team's proposals.

The team had offered a broad plan and an opportunity to impose the rigours of commercial life onto the NHS, without the political fall out of a more root and branch change. The providers of care, not least the powerful body of health professionals, would be directly managed and made to respond to both central Government requirements and, allegedly, to the direct demands of the consumers. A new commercial style with financial rewards and punishments would provide the much needed push to set the show firmly onto the road and to make progress possible. Rather than the previously guaranteed source of financial allocations, the new approach was about payment for proven outcomes and successes – not least that of pleasing the consumer and gaining value for money.

All in all, according to Flynn, Williams & Pickard (1986):

> *The logic which drove these changes was the axiomatic belief that markets were the most efficient means of allocating resources and of reflecting consumer preferences, and therefore market mechanisms should be applied to public services to improve their performance, to control their budgets, and to make them more conscious of clients and users.*

This professed belief in the centrality of the consumer voice in health care delivery was to be continued and developed still further by the introduction of the internal health care market in April 1991. This, together with the managerial changes which had developed since 1984, created the broad backcloth of reform against which we can begin to judge just how much more power the consumers of health care have really achieved.

The creation of the internal health care market: 1989 and onwards

As we have discussed in an earlier chapter, the outcome of the debates of the 1988 review of the health service was published in the 1989 White Paper 'Working for Patients' (Cmd 555 1989). The NHS was to remain a publicly resourced organisation, with the provision of health services (Directly Managed Units (DMUs), community and hospital trusts, general practices, private sector) separated from the purchasing bodies, (private patients, health authorities, and GP budget holders). This internal health care market was to be created to produce greater efficiency and increased quality of care through the use of competition between provider bodies. The managerial developments and lessons learnt from the commercial sector post Griffiths (Griffiths 1983) would oil the wheels of change. According to Flynn, Williams & Pickard (1996):

> *A central thread running through the rhetoric of reform has been that greater managerial control over professional work and enhanced provider competition in the provision of services will give consumers more choice and more control.*

The initial principles underpinning the NHS of 1948 were reaffirmed, that of: comprehensiveness, universality and equity, with efficiency and greater choice for patients as added principles. Some likened the package of reforms to the beginnings of a privatised health system (Cook 1989), something like in the USA (Cairns-Berteau 1991). However, while many on the political right were delighted that such an overhaul was taking place, others were still looking to developing even more complex changes and the creation of a true market oriented service. Whatever their future potential, the consumer, it was claimed, was to be the central focus for all activity within the internal health care market.

Clearly, initial responses to the White Paper of 1989 were mixed and reflected a broad spectrum of ideological and political perspectives. While it was claimed that the consumer was to be the central focus of all activity, others doubted the genuineness of this commitment, and whether the reforms merely represented a clever use of words obscuring other policy objectives which were incompatible with true consumer choice. Perhaps a judgement, on the success or not of the promised focus, might be reached by comparing those concerns expressed by users of the NHS before the changes, with some of the post-reform comment on NHS consumer activity.

Users' concerns – a case to answer?

In September 1989 a consortium of user groups set out a list of worries about the NHS which they wished to see addressed (Voluntary Organisations 1989). The problems highlighted by them included:

◆ Fragmentation of health services between hospitals, community services and general practitioners.

◆ Poor coordination between health and local authority services so that it is easy for people to slip through the gaps.

◆ Inequality of access to health services, both in different geographical areas and for particular disadvantaged groups, such as people from ethnic minorities and homeless people.

◆ Lack of protection and safeguards for patients, such as in making complaints and seeking redress.

◆ Lack of public and community involvement in decision making and planning.

◆ Underfunding of health services, particularly community care.

Any reform of the NHS, they argued, needed to address these problems, but they doubted that this would happen. They felt that many users of the health service who were disadvantaged (e.g. those with physical disabilities, mental health problems, learning difficulties, problem drug and alcohol users and the homeless) were likely to have greater problems after the implementation of the health service changes than before. They perceived that the introduction of competition, even of a managed variety, into the NHS was likely to throw up winners and losers. The losers they felt would probably be the most vulnerable users of the health services. It is clear that these users had many well-thought-out concerns needing attention. We now need to look at some of the debate which has followed the changes, in order to assess the success or not of the reforms, in empowering the consumers of the service.

THE CONSUMERS AND THE REFORMS: EFFORTS TO EMPOWER

The reforms of the 1990s were clearly intended to have a free market feel about them, and to emphasise the opportunity for individuals to demand and to expect the services they desired. Conversely, those health care providers who failed to meet these demands successfully would lose out financially as potential clients went elsewhere in pursuit of other more appropriate and relevant choices on offer in the wider health care market.

However it is interesting to note that while the language of reforms clearly suggested a sort of market relationship between the purchasers and providers of care, the word consumer was never used in the 1989 White Paper to describe the users of the service. Harrison et al (1989) remarked on its surprising absence, because, as they argued: 'By using the terms "patient" and "consumer" as if they were interchangeable, the document not only suggested a narrow conception of the NHS role; it also lacked a framework within which to identify the full range and potential diversity of consumer interests in the field of health'. Indeed, the title of the White Paper 'Working for Patients' reflected an apparently limited remit of NHS concern, i.e. ill consumers. The well consumer, however defined, presumably was not expected to want or need the service.

Despite the early promises of increased individual consumer power, the reality has been perceived in different ways. According to an NHS Management Executive report in January 1992, the NHS was working better than ever, and the consumers gaining greater benefit than previously (NHSME 1992). Changes in the way the NHS was organised had helped to refocus activities. These were leading to improvements in the quality of care, greater responsiveness to individuals and even better value for money.

However, other commentators at that time told a different story. In Chapter 2 we noted that rationalisation and cutting of services had been very much in public evidence, with hospitals and wards being closed. Surgical activity had been slowed up or stopped, because budgets had run out before the end of the financial year. Services previously available free within the NHS were not then available or had attracted new charges. Such outcomes represented for many, stringent prioritising, ever more overt rationing, and as such a much reduced consumer choice. This result was of course directly opposite to the professed aim of the Government's health changes.

The promise to listen to the consumers' views was also felt to be suspect. Some people believed that far from giving people more say in how their health service was run, the reforms actually gave them less (Plamping & Delamothe 1991). They looked to the marginalisation of community health councils, to the changed composition of health authority membership with little or no local representation, to the non-democratic make-up of self-governing trusts and family health service authority management bodies (Mason 1990, Selincourt 1992). As an editorial in 'The Guardian' put it:

> *The restructuring of the NHS has not been restricted to changing the way the health care is delivered. Just as seriously it has been accompanied by tighter restrictions on the release of information to the public. Under the new scheme, community health councils (CHCs) have been shunted into the sidings, and the new health authorities given far more freedom to shut out the press and the public. The new style authorities have seized on this new chance of secrecy. Medics and consumer representatives are now in a minority; the majority of non-executive members are drawn from industry, business, the law and accountancy. A recent survey showed one out of five was only going to meet in public once a quarter. Two out of three were refusing to allow even community health council representatives to remain in private sessions'. (Editorial 1991)*

Some described the consumerist stance which had emerged as being very limited, all about public relations, but certainly not true consumerism. Mahon (1992), for example, referred disparagingly to the emphasis given to reducing waiting lists, to the chasing of quality care, to reducing costs, and to the improvement of information flows. Although important changes in themselves, she was more concerned at the vagueness of these initiatives, and to how they would translate in practice into greater choice for the consumers in the long term. While we are considering the outcomes in this way, we can profitably return again (with our eye on the consumer angle) to the workings of the internal health care market. This also is apparently not quite as it seems.

Will the real consumers stand up?

It had been said by many commentators that the activity of the internal market in the health service had very little to do with consumer choice. We might consider the fact that in a true market situation the customer is in a direct relationship in terms of buying and choosing a product. This is not true in the NHS. The people who purchase and choose care from the provider bodies are not the real or supposed consumers, but the health authorities and budget-holding GPs who thus wield great power.

In the NHS market place, the purchasing authorities and GP fundholders call the tune, and if the providers do not sing along they may lose their voice altogether. (Willis 1992)

So, as we can see, the purported consumer has not only not been at the forefront of choice making and competition, but in reality represents the currency by which improvements in efficiency and financial control of internal health markets were to be achieved. Hospitals have been funded more directly for the volume of the services they provide, and those hospitals which have offered patients the best service and the best value for money have been better rewarded than those which did not; that is, the notion of money following the patient. Maybe the consumer as a result of changes has benefited, but not it seems as a result of being able to influence change directly.

Another point to consider, as has been suggested by some, is that the real intention of the new internal market mechanism was to make clinicians work within management objectives, to keep costs down and to push up productivity rather than meet patients' preferences (Pollitt 1989). As Griffiths said earlier in the 1980s: 'Clinicians must participate fully in decisions about priorities in the use of resources', (Griffiths 1983). This theme was further developed in the White Paper (Cmd 555 1989). 'The decisions taken by consultants are critical to the way in which the money available for the NHS is used. It is therefore important to ensure that consultants are properly accountable for the consequences of these decisions'. The reforms set out proposals for striking a proper balance between two legitimate pressures, both of which were focused on patients' interests: the professional responsibilities and rewards of the individual consultants, and the responsibility of managers to ensure that the money available for hospitals buys the best possible service for patients. Again the benefits of this have been perceived as improving the service to consumers, but in no way has the consumer been a participant involved in influencing directly any change in the amount of NHS funding monies made available – rather consumers have been seen as the recipients of others' decisions and priorities. The internal market so created seems to have been a structure not primarily designed to empower clients directly.

If, as it appears, the consumer is no more powerful now than previous to the changes, perhaps one might consider the inevitability of this occurrence. As already described, the collectivist NHS came into being to overcome the vagaries of failure of a market provision in health care. Why should a partial return to a market-like situation be any more successful in the 1990s? Indeed, if we also agree with Aneurin Bevan's stated beliefs that the NHS he helped to create could never meet all the needs of all the people either (Foot 1973), then are we now all chasing and hoping for some illusory notion of absolute choice? The Conservative Government, however, did not appear to believe or even to acknowledge such an idea. While promising greater choice and power from the internal market reforms introduced to the NHS, the Government, with much publicity, armed the consumers with what some have described as a paper chase of charters.

The charters – frills and trappings?

The charters were intended to set standards against which the public, the professionals and the politicians could check care and treatment provided by public bodies. Supposedly they would enable people to demand good quality care.

In the foreword to the Citizen's Charter, for example (Cmd 1599 1991), John Major, the then Prime Minister, wrote about making public services more answerable to their users and raising their overall quality. He saw this as part of a wider reform programme started in the 1980s which included schools, housing and health care. Four key words exemplified his plans to give people more say in how their services were run:

◆ Quality.
◆ Standards.
◆ Choice.
◆ Value.

If the consumers of the services were not happy with any of these aspects they could just go elsewhere.

These ideas were reiterated in 'The Patient's Charter', (Department of Health 1991), to put power in the hands of the public by highlighting for the first time their rights within the reformed health service. It created standards by which the health care user could assess the performance of any provider body. However, they were described as: 'Not legal rights, but major and specific standards which the Government looks to the NHS to provide as circumstances allow'. (Department of Health 1991).

Kargar (1993), however, was dismissive of the power of the Charters to ensure better health care and choice for consumers. Winkler's description (Winkler 1987) of NHS activity as a 'supermarket model of consumerism' fits in aptly with another's description of the Charter as 'the frills and trappings of patient power' (Editorial 1991). The shopping analogies which emerged time after time seem sadly particularly apt. It seems that the Charters are a bit like the free gifts offered by retailers – they are an encouragement to buy, but not to create the product on the shelf. Some would argue they could be seen as merely representing a cynical ploy to give the public an image of power, but little weight in reality.

An examination on the 'man in the street's' views by a nurse journal reporter, a year after the publication of 'The Patient's Charter' found that:

The concept of patient's rights was largely endorsed, but appeared to remain theoretical. There was widespread cynicism about whether these so-called rights were anything more than paper promises, intended more for public show than for real change. (Nursing Times 1992)

Indicators and information

In a similar vein, the publication of indicators comparing hospital performances has been introduced (Agnew 1995). It was suggested that they were to provide the public with information about which hospital is better than another, and presumably to help make choices about where to go for treatment (Nursing Times 1995). Moon & Lupton (1995) and others, however, have concluded that all of this; whether charter standards, hospital indicators or the wide consultation of consumer views by health authority and other internal market bodies, have all been more above providing information for the market and for those involved in contracting, rather than in empowering the users and giving them a choice. Decisions about movement between hospitals, and responses to standards reached (good or bad), have remained with the purchaser bodies: the health authorities and fundholder practices. While the contracting processes of the internal health care market clearly gave both voice and choice to others, the users still potentially had another avenue to use their power – that of making complaints.

Making complaints – being heard

The Wilson Committee was set up in 1993 by the then Health Secretary, Virginia Bottomley, to examine ways of improving complaints procedures as part of the Government's commitment to taking forward 'The Patient's Charter' and to empowering further the users of the service. As she said in a letter accompanying the completed report (Bottomley 1994):

I want to make sure that the National Health Service, which provides health care to millions of people each year, makes it easy for people to say what they think about its services. (Bottomley 1994)

In the report Wilson acknowledged that complaining is an important way in which patients, families, friends and carers make their views known to the NHS. However, he also believed that it was by no means easy to raise concerns. As he explained:

They (the users) are not in a powerful position and may feel vulnerable. The response they get when they make a complaint is a fundamental test of the NHS as a public service. (Wilson 1994)

The proposals within the report recommended a number of principles which needed to underpin the complaints procedures, and against which NHS managers and others involved in health care delivery should check their progress – not least in responding to the needs and wishes of the users. Complaints procedures, it was suggested, needed to be accessible, well publicised, simple to understand and use, allow speedy handling within reasonable time limits, ensure a full and impartial investigation, and demonstrate respect for people's wishes for confidentiality.

The clarification of the complaints procedures in the NHS which followed has, on the face of it, potentially strengthened the consumer voice, not least judging by the rising levels of complaints since 1994 (Department of Health 1995).

Of course, these complaints may reflect a number of interlinking issues, some of which will be revisited in other chapters:

◆ Dissatisfaction with the service.
◆ Insufficient funding of the service to meet the expressed needs of the users.
◆ Raised expectations of users backed up by the Charter promises to meet their needs.

While the structures for complaining may have been elucidated, many would still acknowledge implicit difficulties for some users. A continuing lack of knowledge and understanding of the complaints system, together with an inability to make progress with a complaint, is unsurprising. Although offering an illusion of power for all, the reality, as we have noted, is often something very different in practice.

A JUDGEMENT SO FAR

So, has the reformed model of NHS care, backed by its charters and so full of promises, really offered users something better than before? We need to keep in mind that the true health care consumer should surely be offered a wide variety of options, to be kept fully informed and involved in managing their care. The reader should reflect on the concerns of the user groups noted earlier, and also think about their own experiences, and decide whether the reforms have facilitated the improvements sought. Inevitably conclusions will be mixed.

Many nurses of course will rightly defend the efforts they have made in recent years to give better care, and to give users a stronger voice in negotiating that care. They will look to developments in both the role and practice of nurses, and to increasing sensitivity and ability in providing individualised care. They will look to work on quality assurance as a way of demonstrating a genuine concern for patient's interests and upholding standards of care. All of these examples should be applauded. However, the issue of promoting a true consumerist approach in the NHS surely involves a much wider remit than the apparent 'window-dressing' and 'frills and trappings' approach being offered via the reforms. According to Mahon (1992), any new development in client behaviour and expectation is going to take longer than a few years, and to need more than a new name to become in reality something significantly different. This, according to Mahon, would require a shift away from the harmless version of consumerism achieved so far, towards alternative models that explore the nature of the doctor–nurse–patient relationship and embrace the concepts of involvement, empowerment and advocacy. Such a shift would require radical changes in the institutional and cultural context of health service provision. We surely have to acknowledge that such moves are not something which have been actively sought in recent years in the NHS.

THE 1997 GENERAL ELECTION: COURTING THE ELECTORATE

By the end of 1996, and in preparation for the General Election of 1997, the Conservative Government published its views on the future of the NHS. The White Paper 'The National Health Service: a service with ambitions' (Cmd 3425 1996) highlighted the continued focus on the users of the service. As Dorrell said in the foreword:

In an increasingly complex and sophisticated service we need to ensure that the patient's interest continues to be the driving force of the whole system. The Government recognises these changes, and believes that the NHS must also be responsive, a service which is sensitive to the needs and wishes of patients and carers.

The objectives of his vision for the NHS included:

◆ A well-informed public.
◆ A seamless service.
◆ Knowledge-based decision making.
◆ A highly trained and skilled workforce.
◆ A responsive service, sensitive to differing needs.

No doubt, Griffiths a decade and more earlier, would have applauded the essence of this missions statement; in addition, no one could deny the remarkable degree of change within the management and organisational structures of the NHS since the Inquiry Team's investigations in 1983.

A different picture however was presented by the Labour Party in opposition during this pre-election period. Chris Smith, then Shadow Secretary of

State for Health, reflected back over the same period that we have covered in the discussion and concluded:

Despite the outstanding support the public gives to the concept of the NHS, the service itself has been slow to harness this support. In many instances it has set up barriers, or hidden behind walls of jargon and expertise and secrecy, which have made it very difficult for people to feel empowered or to have more control over their treatment. Communities, too, have lacked a strong input and stake in the decisions that are made on their behalf. (Smith 1996)

The Labour Party in opposition confirmed three aspects they considered important in the search for the development of a real say for patients and the public in the NHS:

1. Patients' informed decision making about their own treatment.
2. Patients' involvement in shaping services more broadly.
3. Citizens' involvement in determining how the NHS is run.

In conclusion Smith said:

The market-driven changes brought in by the Tories have increased, not decreased the distance between the NHS and the public it serves. Our aim in Government will be to bring the public and Health Service closely together, involved with each other, to the benefit of both.

The election of the Labour Government in May 1997 provided such a chance.

THE NEW NHS. MODERN. DEPENDABLE' (CMD 3807 1997)

Central to all of the proposed changes envisaged in the White Paper was the removal of the lingering and negative effects of the internal health care market – not least the lack of a true focus on the needs and preferences of the users. By contrast, the new way would involve a rebuilding of public confidence in the NHS as a public service, one which was accountable, open to the public and shaped by their views. The ending of the climate of commercial secrecy and the withholding of information from the public was an important theme. The re-energising of public interest and involvement was set out very clearly:

The new arrangements need to be transparent so that they command public confidence. The government expects Health Authorities to play a strong role in communicating with local people and ensuring public involvement in decision-making about the local health service. The NHS, as a public service for local communities should be both responsive and accountable. Health Authorities will need to:

◆ *involve the public in developing the Health Improvement Programme*
◆ *ensure that Primary Care Groups have effective arrangements for public involvement*
◆ *participate in a new national survey of patient and user experience. (4.19)*

The rebuilding of public confidence in NHS trusts was also proposed in the White Paper.

The Government will make NHS Trusts more open and accountable. Action has been taken to ensure that NHS Trusts hold their meetings in public and that Board membership is more representative of the local community. To buttress these changes, no management information in the future will be classified as 'commercial in confidence' between NHS bodies. Such a classification is simply not appropriate for organisations that are publicly funded and accountable, and are expected to operate as trusted partners working together to the common goal of better health and healthcare for local people. (6.39)

As part of its rolling programme of modernisation underpinned by user partnerships, the Government also promised to ensure that the experience of users and carers is fed into both new NHS developments and into the evaluation of the outcomes of treatment and care given.

As part of the new framework, the Government will take special steps to ensure the experience of users and carers is central to the work of the NHS. The current Patient's Charter was introduced without adequate consultation and concentrated too much on narrow measures of process. A New NHS Charter will therefore be developed in partnership with NHS users and carers and the staff of the service. It will place greater emphasis on the outcomes of treatment and care. It will focus on things that really matter. (8.9)

The Government has said that the health service would now begin to measure itself against the aspirations and experiences of its users. A new annual national survey of patient and user experience would be introduced, with the results published both locally and nationally. It is suggested that this survey will give patients and their carers a voice in shaping the NHS. The first survey would take place in 1998. (8.10)

As far as the future is concerned, the Government has promised to work with the user in a different and maybe stronger way than hitherto. Clearly, the success and effectiveness of the proposed initiatives remain to be seen.

However, the enthusiasm for greater openness and the importance clearly given to the views of the users, together with the constructive initiatives proposed, are suggestive of a more positive approach.

AN AGENDA FOR NURSES: THE CHALLENGE FOR THE FUTURE

The discussion so far has come to the following broad conclusions. In many respects the previous Conservative governments' emphasis and language have put the health care consumer onto the agenda in a more pronounced way than at any other time in the history of the NHS. On the other hand, it is felt that the consumer participation offered has been limited and, at best, indirect. It is in this contradiction that both a challenge and a risk emerge for nurses. As with 'apple pie and motherhood', everyone is going to be in favour of increased consumer choice. Nurses will be no exception, as professional values and modern practice both point in the same direction of greater negotiation between nurse and patient, and greater choice on the part of the patient.

If it is accepted, as argued in the earlier part of this chapter, that the previous Government's programme for the NHS did not add greatly to consumer choice, and, indeed with the introduction of market values and disciplines and stringent resourcing may have made access to health care more socially unequal, then the agenda of consumer choice assumes a more radical dimension. Nurses, and their organisations, which argue that there is a link between effective consumer choice and adequate resourcing, will be faced with the task of participating in all those debates around the sufficiency and redistribution of resources within the NHS. Perhaps that is the only route if nurses are to speak with strength and conviction on behalf of their clients, and in turn help them to become empowered users of the service. They are then by desire or by implication moving into a more sharply defined political agenda. The question remains therefore whether nursing as a profession is confident enough in itself to try and achieve such an objective.

REFERENCES

Abel-Smith B 1976 Value for money in health services. Heinemann, London
Agnew T 1995 League tables 'bad for staff morale'. Nursing Times. 12 July 91(28): 9
Allsop J 1996 Health policy and the NHS, towards 2000. Longman, London
Benzeval M, Judge K, Whitehead M 1995 Tackling inequalities in health. King's Fund, London
Black D 1980 Inequalities in health. Report of a research working group. HMSO, London
Bottomley V 1994 In: Wilson A. Being heard. Department of Health, London
Butler J 1992 Patients, policies and politics. Open University Press, Milton Keynes
Cairns-Berteau M 1991 LA Flaw. Nursing Times 87(5): 36–38
Cook R 1989 Statement NHS Review. Hansard 146(39) 165–189

Command 249 1987 Promoting Better Health. Department of Health, London

Command 555 1989 Working for Patients. Department of Health, London

Command 1599 1991 The Citizen's Charter. HMSO, London

Command 3425 1996 The National Health Service: a service with ambitions. Department of Health, London

Command 3807 1997 The New NHS. Modern. Dependable. Department of Health, London

Department of Health 1991 The Patient's Charter. Department of Health, London

Department of Health 1995 Written complaints by or on behalf of patients. 1993–1994. Department of Health, London

Donaldson L 1995 The listening blank. Health Service Journal 25 September, pp 22–24

Dorling D 1997 Death in Britain: how local mortality rates have changed: 1950s–1990s

Editorial 1991 Stealthy is not very healthy. The Guardian. 20 May

Editorial 1991 Comment. Nursing Times 87(45): 3

Fatchett A 1994 Politics. Policy and nursing. Baillière Tindall, London

Flynn R, Williams G, Pickard S 1996 Markets and networks. Contracting in community health services. Open University Press, Milton Keynes

Foot M 1973 Aneurin Bevan, vol 2. Davis Poynter, London

Griffiths R 1983 The NHS management inquiry report. DHSS, London

Harrison S, Hunter D, Johnston I, Wistow G 1989 Competing for health: a commentary on the NHS review. Nuffield Institute Reports, University of Leeds

Kargar I 1993 Charter of charters. Nursing Times 89(2): 22

Klein R 1980 Models of man and models of policy. Milbank Memorial Fund, London

Klein R 1989 The politics of the NHS. 2nd edn. Longman, London

Mahon 1992 Feature. Manchester University patient survey. Health Service Journal. 3 December

Mason P 1990 Consumers' voice. Nursing Times. 86(31): 20–21

Moon G, Lupton C 1995 Within acceptable limits: health care provider perspectives on Community Health Councils in the reformed National Health Service. Policy and Politics. 23: 335–346

NHSME National Health Service Management Executive 1992 NHS Reforms: the first six months. HMSO, London

Normand 1991 Economics, health and the economics of health. British Medical Journal. 303: 1572–1577

North N, Bradshaw Y (eds) 1997 Perspectives in health care. Macmillan, Basingstoke

Nursing Times 1992 Power to the people. 89(14): 32–33

Nursing Times 1995 NHS league tables out this week. 90(26): 6

Plamping D, Delamothe T 1991 The Citizen's Charter and the NHS. British Medical Journal 303: 203–204

Pollitt C 1989 Consuming Passions. Health Service Journal. 99(5178): 1436–1437

Potter J 1988 Consumerism and the public sector. How well does the coat fit? Public Administration. 66: 149–164

Pyne R 1992 Changing the code. Nursing Times 88(25): 20–22

Schultz R, Harrison S 1983 Teams and top managers in the NHS: a survey and a strategy. Project paper no 41. Kings Fund, London

De Selincourt K 1992 Power to the patients. Nursing Times. 88(33): 18

Sheldon A (ed) 1980 The Litmuss Papers. Centre for Policy Studies, London

Smith C 1996 (MP – Shadow Health Secretary) A health service for a new century – Labour's proposals to replace the internal market in the NHS. 3 December

United Kingdom Central Council 1992 Code of professional conduct for the nurse, midwife and health visitor, 3rd edn. UKCC

Voluntary Organisation 1989 Health services users and the NHS review. A statement from voluntary organisations. London

Willis J 1992 The price of health. Nursing Times. 88(30): 24–26

Wilson A 1994 Being heard. Department of Health, London

Winkler F 1987 Consumerism in health care: beyond the supermarket model. Policy and Politics 15(1): 1–8

6

Nursing and professional development

◆ *Nurses in Europe are not a homogenous group: large differences are found in the roles they play, the tasks they perform, the training they receive, the status they have in society and the remuneration they get for their work. Taken together, however, they comprise a formidable workforce that provides some of the most essential services to keep people healthy, to take care of the ill and the injured, and to nurse the frail and elderly throughout the region.*

◆ *In many, if not most, European countries, these health professionals unfortunately do not get the recognition they deserve, or the working facilities they need to carry out their unique function in our health care systems.*

(Asvall 1997; WHO Regional Director for Europe)

Asvall's comments very much reflect the general tenor of the two main themes which underpin the discussion to follow. On the one hand, attention will be given to nursing's attempts over time to achieve the status and rewards of a full profession within the National Health Service (NHS) . On the other hand, it will be suggested that this goal has been both illusory and probably inappropriate – evidenced by the difficult challenges and changes which British nurses have faced during a period of NHS reform.

In order then to facilitate the exploration of a number of detailed and interlinking issues the discussion will take the following route:

1. The NHS reforms: challenges to nurse professionalism.
2. The concept of professionalism.
3. Nurses as professionals: debates and developments over time.
4. Professionalism under threat:
   – the impact of general management;
   – the NHS internal market reforms.
5. Agenda for nurse professionalism.
6. Whistleblowing.
7. Pay, casualisation and skill mixing.
8. The future for professional nursing.

THE NHS REFORMS: CHALLENGES TO NURSE PROFESSIONALISM

The role of the professional nurse, associated values and achievements have been seriously challenged during the period of internal market reform. While many nurses have indeed thrived and created positive niches for themselves (Fatchett 1998), and are now well prepared to take up new opportunities, others inevitably have been unable to survive the demands made upon them (Gillan 1994, Thornton 1995). Perhaps no one should be too surprised at such an outcome. The positive claims made for the reforms which were designed to have benefited the users, the service and professional nurses alike, have not always lived up to expectations. In earlier chapters, for example, it has been argued that the creation of the internal health care market and increased commercialisation of NHS activity have not improved the services for all.

Health care inequalities, for instance, have widened during the period of reform (Benzeval, Judge & Whitehead 1995). Health care consumers have not been further empowered (Donaldson 1995), but merely offered a 'window dressing' of choice. The avowed intent to make the NHS more concerned with the promotion of good health has also been questioned because of the emphasis on secondary care (Haggard 1995). The often stated support and enthusiasm for effective multidisciplinary collaboration in care has been made even more difficult by the creation of competitive and fragmented structures within the NHS, together with the development of its more commercialised approach. The process of implementing the market mechanisms and the underpinning contract culture have been antipathetic to good collaborative initiatives (Nocon 1994). In turn, the apparent redefinition of the concept of need, and what may be construed as the focus of NHS business, have resulted in the continuing development of a service which is focused on secondary and tertiary care and medical services – in spite of many assertions to the contrary. Indeed, in relation to the meeting of assessed need and the promised empowerment of the users of the service, there is a great deal left to be desired (North & Bradshaw 1997). Flaws and cracks have appeared over time in the NHS market environment, which have created uncertainties and inequalities in provision, which have felt sharper and more uncomfortable than they ever did before the changes took place. Professional nurses have not been immune to such feelings as they have continued to work in the rapidly changing and often difficult environment of care.

All nurses will have experienced these uncomfortable developments to some degree or other. Gough (1997), for example, described the health reforms as a stunning case study of the marginalisation of the nursing contribution. Many indeed have felt professionally compromised during this period, because of their inability to respond as fully as they may have wished to the assessed needs of their clients. Others (Mangan 1983, Allsop 1995) have reflected on the impacts of the marketised approach to health care delivery, with its primary emphasis on the measurement of costs, contract making and money flows. A secondary interest has been shown in the apparently peripheral qualitative concepts around service to the client, or indeed for this discussion to nurse professional growth and development. Meehan (1996) observed that:

> . . . *nursing care was being sacrificed on the high altar of finance as nursing posts were being shed left, right and centre in a desperate attempt by health care trusts to balance the books.*

As such, the past years of reform have not been easy for professional nurses. However, this is an unsurprising observation. Nurses are, and always have been, central players in the NHS. There is no way that they could have been above or removed from the various outcomes already noted. The impact of the managerial and market culture has without doubt controlled and shaped the extent to which nurse professional development has been encouraged and afforded. After all, high status professionals are expensive to employ in great numbers, and it is easy to see how the creation of a more flexible, less powerful and cheaper care workforce has held an obvious appeal to cost-conscious managers.

The expressions of doubt as to the need to employ professional nurses were very evident in the early 1990s (Caines 1993, Dyson 1993). These concerns have been matched lately by the development of the support worker role (Fatchett 1996), the upskilling of cleaners to care for the elderly, terminally ill, (Goodchild 1995, Leifer 1996), the use of robots to deliver records and samples (Brown 1996), questionnaires to replace health visitors (Kenny 1997a) and health promotion leaflets to replace school nurses (Kenny 1997b) Finally, a proposal has been made that serious consideration should be given to the replacement of the professional nurse role by that of a generic carer – a broader-based carer role, encompassing the responsibility for coordinating patient care and delivering most of it in the NHS of the future (Manchester University 1996).

Responses to the last proposed development were, unsurprisingly, polarised. Caines (1996) argued that it was time to scrap the boundaries between doctors and nurses and to create a simple clinical group. Everybody could undertake the same basic health care training, but would progress as far as individual inclinations or aptitudes permitted. Further to this, Conroy (1996), project director of the research, argued that tinkering with the current range of health care roles was not enough, and that the changes proposed would allow employers to plan what staff they wanted around patient needs and the work to be done, rather than based on traditional role demarcations. Her team's solution was the creation of a flexible workforce, the centre point of which would be a 'generic health practitioner responsible for continuity of care'. An additional point of importance was that the then (in 1996) 28% of support workers contributing to nursing care work should be expanded to 40% by 2010. The two other main staff groups would be technicians, and a combination of doctors, therapists and scientists. In response to these proposals, the NHS Executive, who had commissioned the work, called the report interesting and well researched, adding that the more radical conclusions would need more careful considerations (Agnew 1996).

However, responses from health professionals in general, and nursing in particular, were explosive. Comments ranged from: 'nonsense' (English 1996), 'out of touch with reality and an unsophisticated response to complex and challenging questions' (Hancock 1996), to 'a cover for managers to cut qualified nursing staff' (Chapman 1996). All of the ideas implicit within the report were seen in combination as yet another potential body blow to the credibility of the nursing profession.

One nurse journal editorial sharply and succinctly stated that nurses wished to remain within their distinctively named and known care profession, and not least if the Government gave them the recognition, authority and tools to do their job properly (Nursing Times 1996). These hard words reflect a strong and very sincerely held defence of nursing's professional role. On this point we will now turn to look more closely at what being a professional means, and why the maintenance of such a status is so very important to all in nursing.

THE CONCEPT OF PROFESSIONALISM

What is a Professional?

In very common usage the term professional is seen as a collective symbol of high value (Becker 1970), often implying dedication and commitment. However, from the vast expanse of literature on it, there emerges a multitude of definitions and perspectives (Hugman 1991, Turner 1991). The analysis of the concept of a professional has been a major preoccupation of sociologists over time (see, for example, Parsons 1939, Durkheim 1951, Weber 1966, Friedson 1970, Johnson 1972). It is evident that like discussions around the concepts of health, need and care, for example, the debates around the nature of professionalism are also complex, sometimes contradictory, and in the end rely upon individual perception, understanding and experience. A brief note, however, on just some of the points raised will help to clarify the discussions to follow.

Durkheim (1951), for example, looked to the professional groups as representing an institutionalisation of personal service and community welfare. Weber (1966) described professionals as motivated by neither personal interests nor economic reward. Parsons (1939, 1951) emphasised the ethical nature of their work, providing a service to others based on technical knowledge. Mannheim described them as providing a guarantee of objectivity and being above sectional interests (see Turner 1991). Kaye in turn looked to a profession as 'an occupation possessing skilled intellectual technique, a voluntary association and a code of conduct'. He believed that the last factor, the code of conduct, provided 'the guarantee of integrity, that is the main distinguishing mark of the professions' (Kaye 1965). This 'guarantee of integrity' will be referred to later when we examine the issue of whistleblowing and attempts to apply professional codes of conduct where standards of practice or care appear to be compromised in health care settings.

Meanwhile, other views on the nature of professions are also worthy of note. Greenwood (1957) and Millerson (1964) have listed characteristics or traits of professional groups, as follows:

◆ Skills based on theoretical understanding.
◆ Autonomy in judgements.
◆ Tested competence in achieving prescribed standards.
◆ Possession of a service ethic, so that they work for the common good rather than in their own self interest.

As Hugman explains it:

Each occupation to be considered as a candidate for the label professional could be compared to the list of traits, and the degree to which it matched was then taken as an indication of the extent to which the occupation was professional. (Hugman 1991)

Following from this Etzioni (1969) applied the 'trait' approach to nurses, social workers and teachers, and defined them as semiprofessionals, because he found them to be highly managed and controlled within their working environments. In addition, their work, he suggested, lacked specific (to them) theoretical underpinning and emphasised skills rather than knowledge. By comparison, medicine and law, for example, had a greater claim to professional status than nursing. In yet another perspective, professionalism is seen as a form of occupational control (Friedson 1970, Johnson 1972). In this way the profession decides who should or should not belong, for instance, in nursing through the use of state registration. In this way a qualified nurse, for example, is acknowledged to be a safer and more knowledgeable practitioner than someone who is not. Such self-regulation is very common amongst health carers throughout the world (Peters et al 1978). The specialist knowledge and skills acquired by members enable them to a greater or lesser degree to claim autonomy in judgements about their care, and to be free from management and supervision. In reality of course, the ability of any health care professional to wield total power or control over their work is constrained by others. This is likely to involve members of the same profession, other allied professions, those who are paying for the care, the consumers or users of the services, and wider social institutions, for example, acting on behalf of the Government. By these means, the content and activity of professional care, in whatever sphere, are determined both within and without, and between professions. The power relationships thus created are obviously complex, with all sides seeking to achieve their own ends by both overt and covert means. Suffice it to say, all professional groups within the NHS have not been immune from such processes during their development.

Professionals in the NHS

The NHS is crammed with professionals. They would all to a greater or lesser degree subscribe to a traditional vision of their role: the notion of having operational autonomy, a concern with giving service immediately to a client in need, and a belief that their specialist knowledge and skills can only be provided by members of their particular profession. Indeed, they must by definition see themselves as protecting the public from outsiders; for example, from unscrupulous practitioners who have been expelled from their professional body, from quacks, amateurs and unscientific methods. It is no wonder then that any group would wish to be acknowledged as a profession, and to have the opportunity to shape their practice and to garner good financial rewards in the process. According to Heller (1978), the medical profession could be said to have achieved such professional status and power within the NHS. Nurses, however, have clearly been less successful in this quest. They have failed to achieve control over their practice, with their autonomy and power clearly circumscribed by managerial hierarchies.

Nurses as professionals

The debate around whether or not nurses are professionals is often hot and full of fury, with one branch asserting its predominance of attributes over another. While Watkins (1992) refers to health visiting and midwifery as professions, he states that nursing:

> *lacks the key attributes of a profession, its members are not mutually supportive; they do not seek to control their own work, it does not have high expectations of its working conditions, its brightest and ablest members are not the ones who rise within it.*

Another commentator (McEvoy 1992) refers to 'nursing as not yet exhibiting the full characteristics of a profession, but as soundly established on the continuum'. He and others (see Bridges 1991) note a variety of ways in which progress had been made, for example with the creation of professional organisations, the development of an international code of ethics, the development of conceptual frameworks for practice, the creation of degree courses in nursing and the emergence of nursing research upon which to base practice.

In spite of such positive progress, Watkins notes 'the dead hand of nursing attitudes' which halt those who wish to make greater professional strides than others. In this context he cites those nurses who side with obstetricians against midwives who seek independent practitioner status. While clearly not referring to this midwifery example, Rundell (1991) notes in a similar vein that:

> *The nursing profession appears happy to defer to its "betters" to avoid its responsibilities, and readily defends the prejudices and bizarre rituals of its colleagues in medicine for the sake of a quiet life.*

Rundell believes that people in general, and nurses in particular, still defer to doctors instead of valuing nursing as a profession every bit as skilled and valuable as medicine. However, this is hardly surprising, because of the historical closeness of nursing to medicine. It is perhaps because of the long-time pursuit of, and adherence to the medical knowledge base and values, that nursing has failed to achieve the status and power as a distinct profession with its own theory base and *raison d'être*.

Another anti-professionalising attitude among nurses is the commonly held belief that nurses have to be all things to all people to prove that they are good professionals. Surely, however, to develop as a profession, nursing needs good managers, good educators, good practitioners, good researchers, good politicians and good writers. Other professions would expect no less. As Watkins (1992) stated:

> *Most professions advance their most able members; nurses treat colleagues who advance to the top as dysfunctional: a nurse who moves into management is either seen to have "failed" as a nurse or is not a true nurse. (see Faugier 1992, Shelley 1993)*

Indeed, any nurse who tries to take a stand for nursing is often vilified and left isolated, because occupational solidarity in nursing has been historically poor. While doctors will support their own and have very powerful professional representative organisations, nurse organisations too often seem to be in competitive bidding for members on the one hand, while on the other, fiercely defending status hierarchies in a way which makes it impossible to have collaboration with other groups of NHS employees (see Murray 1990 on the ambulance dispute, Cohen 1993). Sadly, these internal arguments may also be sapping important energies which could be used elsewhere to better effect in the pursuit of a professional role. It has been said that nurses often fail to appreciate the power of wider societal factors which determine the context within which nursing is carried out, and which in turn define the status and content of nurse work. According to Robinson (1991), the inequalities which are seen in society as a whole are reflected in the nursing workforce. The exploitation of women in the wider society is thus recreated in health care settings. As Gamarnikow (1978) has explained:

Women are exploited as nurses because they are socialised into a doctrine which associates nursing with mothering, and sees the hospital ward as merely an expansion of the domestic sphere of labour.

In this way 'the good women' (Nightingale 1881), or 'housewives of medicine' (Gamarnikow 1978), who carry out the nursing role, are apparently tied into a socially constructed picture of formally carrying out women's work. This in turn has had the effect of legitimising the lower status given to nurse caring, particularly in relation to the care given by those in the medical and allied scientific professions, (see Game & Pringle 1983, Oakley 1984).

Salvage (1990) acknowledges the many efforts made by nurses to challenge these prevailing images, which serve to downgrade nurse care by implying that it is natural and intuitive women's work, rather than an occupation, predominately composed of women, who are involved with giving care of a professional nature. She would like to see a much greater emphasis placed by nurses on the analysis, understanding and response to the wider and fundamental societal issues about power and gender. For in the end, society's attitude to women and women's work is central to the vision and worth it ascribes to nurses and nursing, and as such to its professional credibility.

Sadly, nursing as an occupational group has spent more time historically contemplating itself and its internal strategies within the health service. This without a doubt has promoted important theoretical developments, improved understanding and advanced practice in line with new health care needs. However, according to Witts (1992), modern definitions of what nursing is all about are 'both numerous and diverse' and continue to 'reflect the relationship of nursing as a jack-of-all trades support system to medicine and its allied occupations'. It would appear that in spite of internal effort by nurses to grow and develop as professionals alongside medicine, it has largely failed. It does appear that persistent attention to internal strategies alone are unlikely to alter the root causes of nurse professional subordination to the medical profession.

Etzioni's (1969) semiprofessional notion then may well be a fair reflection of the less secure professional base on which nursing stands. Nonetheless, even as a semiprofession, nurses are seen as knowledgeable and are well respected by the general public. Sadly, however, it is suggested that this is only as a result of their long term working relationship with doctors. As Bridges (1991) said 'One reason for the continued use of the medical model for nursing is the high value placed by society on biological survival, resulting in a high status for those disciplines associated with medicine.' Again, this adherence to the medical profession and the metaphorical 'rubbing of shoulders', while providing a halo effect, does not address the disparity in status between doctors and nurses, and how the balance might be changed. It merely reinforces the dependent position of nursing to medicine, and does not encourage a truly collegiate relationship between the groups, which offer complementary, but different caring roles in society. So it would appear that nursings' efforts over time to become a full profession, like medicine, have not succeeded.

Attempts to professionalise the role by developing in-depth knowledge, expanding the scope of practice, expertise and specialisation, and by the shedding of non-nursing work (sterilisation of instruments, preparation of dressings, domestic work and clerical duties), all have apparently been to little avail. By comparison, similar moves to specialisation by doctors have met with much more effective outcomes (Heller 1978). Why should this be so? Why does medicine still continue to hold and develop its professional status, even after the antiprofessional managerial influences of the past decade?

NURSES AS PROFESSIONALS: DEBATES AND DEVELOPMENTS OVER TIME

The apparent failure by nursing to achieve professional credibility in spite of great efforts is unsurprising to Davies (1995). She has described her sense of the inhospitable terrain on which nurses have struggled in recent years and that protests that they were a profession and should be treated as one, seem to have fallen regularly on deaf ears (Davies 1996a). Major reasons for this, she believed, related to the traditional and masculine defined models of professionalism which have been used as benchmarks over time, not least in relation to the predominantly male medical profession, (Davies 1996b). The concept of professionalism as applied to medicine has reflected stereotypical male traits such as: competitiveness, detachment from care, independence in decision making, control and rationality. These are traits which are generally in contrast to and antipathetic to the reflective, attached, caring, interdependent nature of professional nurse care today – in the main carried out by women. Davies proposes the creation of a new, more inclusive model of professionalism, one which values the collection of a more appropriate group of professional carer traits, ones which better reflects the changing nature of user health needs in the late twentieth century and which are relevant to the current developing NHS care delivery systems and organisation.

As she puts it:

Nursing should construct a new model of professionalism that reflects the changing relationships between providers and users, doctors and nurses, and men and women. This revitalised understanding of ourselves is essential if we are to respond creatively to health challenges. (Editorial 1996)

While nursing is thus offered a constructive and exciting objective to pursue, the reality is that any fundamental change of understanding around the concept of professionalism is not likely to be achieved in the near future. Indeed, some may well argue, that 'changing the goalposts' is no way to achieve professional status either. In any event, this particular debate will need to be continued by all nurses for some time to come if nursing is ever to take on the coveted title of a full profession, however defined.

Having said that, whatever definitions are in the ascendancy and whatever their appropriateness or not, nursing as a whole will need to continue to give great attention to two important aspects. First, it should develop further its understanding around those external political forces which shape society's attitudes to women and women in work. Second, nursing will at the same time need to establish ever more strongly its own mission in terms of professional caring, and to explain it to others more clearly than hitherto. In this way, status could be given to the role of professional nurse carers, rather than to that of assistant to medical practice.

Admittedly, this is not likely to be an easy task, judging by what we have seen so far in this chapter. There are those who doubt the need to employ qualified nurses at present levels, and others who view nurses as 'bit players' who should turn their hand to any task or speciality if staffing levels dictate. The support for and promotion of care assistants and support workers, and the proposed development of a generic carer to carry out skilled nursing work, have all served to rebut claims as to the professional nature of nursing care.

While such intellectual self-contemplation and overt political activity are vital to any future successful professionalising agenda for nursing, it is also evident that all nurses need to appreciate and to understand what has been happening to them in the recent past within the NHS. A critical exploration of the background to the situation in which nurses find themselves today, should help to clarify the agendas for professional development which need to be pursued as from tomorrow.

For example, during the whole period of Conservative health reforms some have argued (for example see Ackroyd 1992) that there was a gradual Government-inspired and management-led suppression of the power of health professionals in the NHS. The nursing profession was not immune, and was often under challenge, as were medicine and other allied professions.

It is therefore important to acknowledge the impact of these moves, to avoid any overinflated assessment of the strength of nursing's position as a professional grouping in the NHS of today.

With this in mind, we now look back briefly over a period of almost two decades of changes, and consider how these have restructured the nurse role, and challenged the claim to professional status.

PROFESSIONALISM UNDER THREAT

As already noted, both doctors and nurses have developed their professional roles to a greater or lesser degree. The obvious centrality of their contribution to the workings of a health service have ensured over time both autonomy and great power in the decision-making process. Certainly, in the early 1980s, the professionals had greater power than the managers and administrators. However, the federation inevitable in an organisation as dependent upon professionals as the NHS, meant that there was no single focal point of power or decision making. It was because of this lack of clarity in the management process that the Government determined to introduce a series of changes designed to strengthen NHS management. No group in the health service whether professional or manual was to be left untouched, least of all nurses, in what was to a systematic overhaul of the whole service. Whereas previous governments and their health ministers failed to pursue and hold onto the professional reins, the Conservative governments from 1979 pulled themselves firmly into the driving seat and attempted to make the health care agendas of all professionals and non-professionals alike fall into line.

The impact of general management

For some the introduction of general management in the early 1980s was regarded as an attack both on professional autonomy and clinical freedoms. It thus attracted a predictably hostile reception from both doctors and nurses. However, the Griffiths Inquiry Team (Griffiths 1983) must have expected nothing less. Their specific remit had been to make an assessment of NHS management. It came as no surprise that they concluded that the clear power of professional groups overrode management decision making. The inquiry team had found that the multiplicity of professional role players in the NHS, all demanding that their voice be heard in management circles, led to consensus decisions which were not sharp enough to manage effectively, and also ensured that NHS change was slow and incremental. General management, as in industrial settings, was proposed as a more successful route to take. As in business circles, a knowledge of levels and quality of service, of costs, of employee motivation, of evaluation of services and a commitment to the 'real' consumer of the NHS were needed. All of these proposed changes were presented as the only way of moving forward, to ensure value for money for the taxpayer, together with the provision of an effective and efficient health service which benefited the whole community.

The new management

In the wake of the Griffiths Report, all regional health authorities (RHAs), district health authorities (DHAs) and NHS hospitals (in England) were ordered to appoint general managers by the end of 1985. Together new managers throughout the NHS were to assume responsibility for overall direction and strategic management of the British health care service. A line management funding developed on clear business principles was thereby introduced to the NHS. General managers were mainly in position by 1986 (Holliday 1992), with only 36 of these new-style managers being nurses (Brindle 1993c).

The managers, in the main, plucked from industrial backgrounds, were brought into the NHS to make the necessary changes. Short term contracts, performance-related pay and reviews were introduced to help sharpen their commitment and resolve to deliver the required managerial policies throughout the NHS. While manual workers had already felt the sharp edge of compulsory competitive tendering since 1984, nurses and doctors were now set to feel the impact of a new managerial philosophy which required everyone to come under sharp commercial scrutiny and to prove their worth if they were to stay in business in the NHS.

The nurses – what happened to them?

Elements of the nursing hierarchies were dismantled, including the demise of the traditional matron figures. This in particular represented a rejection of previous professional values with nurses gaining reward for time served in the NHS. In its place came new ideas linking reward and career opportunities to skills, experience and managerial ability. Disappointment was expressed at the low numbers of nurses who became general managers, but then judging from the Griffith's Report, little credence was given to nurses as potential general management material anyway (Spurgeon 1997). Added to all of this, the regrading developments concerning nurse pay in 1987 caused a furore inspiring thousands to take industrial action (Pilkington 1989). In addition to providing an environment of divide and rule between nurses, it opened up wounds which still exist today.

The doctors

Many doctors too felt extremely challenged by the new managerial culture which slipped into the NHS in the mid 1980s – a concern which has continued to reverberate for many (Exworthy 1996, Mihill 1996). That said, in the early days of reform, appeals to the doctors' sense of professional responsibility in serving the public as well as possible, particularly in a period of economic stringency, provided the necessary backcloth to other managerial strategies. Doctors were encouraged to become responsible for clinical budgeting, and to be involved in the use of performance reviews and indicators. All of these enabled management to make comparisons on activity between clinicians. In addition to this, and to oil the wheels of change, improved distinction awards were offered to consultants. Some doctors became general managers. However at that stage others were not convinced by the changes, and held out against them for a long time. Certainly, in these early years, many doctors and nurses continued to try and work as they had done before the introduction of general management, conceding small points to survive. It was clearly obvious to the Government that further reform was needed to develop the required cultural change, and to force the professions into a context in which they had to become a working part of the new business-like NHS or to leave.

The old ways of running a service in which professionals maintained secrecy and thus power in their work was poised to be overthrown even further by the internal market reforms. The managed competition between the purchasers and the providers of the services would both open up and sharpen the delivery of professional practice. Those who delivered 'the business' would benefit financially, as would their employer institution; those who did not would lose out.

As Mangan (1993) said at the time: 'Nurses need to demonstrate their worth if they want to remain as clinicians, teachers and managers in the new NHS' – a theme which sounds uncomfortably familiar even today.

We will now turn to examine the fate of the nursing profession under the internal market reforms.

The NHS internal market reforms

By January 1989 the move to general management, according to the Secretary of State for Health in the White Paper 'Working for Patients', (Cmd 555 1989), was showing results and pointing the way ahead. New management information systems had shown variations in performance up and down the country, different waiting times for care depending on where one lived, and variations in drug prescribing habits and referral rates. For the Secretary of State, professionals of all descriptions could do much better in putting the patients first.

The ways to achieve this laudable objective were set out in the White Paper which Kenneth Clarke, Secretary of State for Health, presented to the House of Commons in January 1989. The details in the Hansard Report are both illuminating and interesting for all nurses (Hansard 1989). A brief look at just some of the points made will be of use to the discussion.

The White Paper debate – the politicians' view (Hansard 1989)

The announcement of the reforms prompted sharp responses from the opposition benches. Robin Cook, Labour Party Shadow Health Secretary, clearly aware of the managerial activity we have discussed, wondered:

> *How many more bureaucrats the NHS will need to make this package work? Will he tell us how much time doctors will have to take off patient care to file their financial returns? Will he tell us how much more the monitoring, the pricing and the bargaining over every treatment will add to the cost of administration, and whether a single closed ward will reopen as a result of this White Paper?*

Cook also queried the lack of discussion with the caring professions involved in the health service. In response Clarke said:

> *There is no reason why the public service should not be run with the same efficiency and consumer consciousness as the private sector – he [Cook] cannot dismiss the value of modern management disciplines, financial accountability and consumer consciousness that we are seeking to build into the health service.*

As far as the lack of consultation with nurses and doctors was concerned, Clarke said that he would talk with them after the publication of a variety of working papers which would provide greater detail of specific changes to be introduced.

As the discussion moved on, one back-bench Labour MP, Michael Foot, again raised the interests of the professions:

> *Will the Right Hon. and learned gentleman now tell us whether he is proposing to have any genuine consultations with people working in the service: with the nurses, the unions, the British Medical Association, and the presidents of the royal colleges?*

Clarke's repudiation of speaking to representative groups only, rather than to all staff, was clear in his response. He stated:

> *The Labour Party's idea of consultation on health policy, as we all know, is to ring up NUPE, reversing the charges, and ask what they should be expected to say. We propose to run the Health Service in an altogether more constructive fashion.*

It would appear then that nurse representative organisations were to be circumvented, and importantly even the largest did not merit mention by name, as they were all lumped together dismissively under NUPE, for fairly obvious reasons. As Audrey Wise, Labour back-bench MP, suggested, the reason why the professions had not been involved in the review in the first place, was that they might have got in the way of the imposition of the changes because they would have disagreed with the whole process. Indeed, Clarke was accused by Dr Lewis Moonie (Labour MP) of only having a tenuous grasp on reality:

> . . . *the proposal is born of the eccentric mind of someone in the Adam Smith Institute who has no concept of what it is like to run a health service, as opposed to talking and thinking about one.*

All in all the parliamentary debates confirmed the feeling that the managerial and market reforms were to be driven through with or without the professionals. None of this, of course, sounded particularly propitious for the development of the nursing profession. Perhaps we need to look for hints within the White Paper itself, so that we can piece together the jigsaw and try to find some answers to our questions around potential nurse professionalism in the post-reform future.

Clues from the White Paper (Cmd 555 1989)

Promises to the nurses from the White Paper included greater satisfaction and rewards for those working in the NHS who successfully respond to local needs and preferences. The Trusts, it said, would harness the skills and dedication of the staff, and would be setting their own conditions, pay rates and rewards for individual performances. A better use of professional staff and their skills was also promised, together with the provision of better training for non-professional support staff. An appraisal of the traditional practices of nurses would result in some doctor tasks being passed to them, and some clerical work taken away. Linked to all of the above was the promise that the nursing profession would become part of resource management initiatives to provide management with more information about nurse care activity and its cost.

Even the initial announcement of the proposed changes and the introduction of market reforms suggested a conflict with the growing professional aspirations of nurses. These concerns have sadly started to be borne out by experience. For example, the pressure to contain costs of NHS spending, the persistent development of the managerial culture and commercialisation, the search for cost-effective clinical effectiveness, a reassessment of skill-mix and possible labour substitutions, and a determined effort to raise the calibre of untrained staff to take on nursing roles, all have clearly contributed to a questioning of the supposed special nature of professional nurse expertise and status – a situation which has continued into the late 1990s.

As was said earlier, professionals perceive they have autonomy in their practice, and by virtue of their superior skills and knowledge know more than other people about what is required to give good, holistic patient care. Backed up by the UKCC Code of Conduct which underpins nurse practice, nurses offer a 'guarantee of integrity' (Kaye 1965), both to those who employ them, and to those who receive their care. That said, the experience of ever-increasing management control over the focus, content and degree of professional nurse care both purchased and provided within the internal health care market has had its effects. In many respects efforts to professionalise nursing through both practice developments and educational change have often felt to be sidelined and ignored, in spite of assertions to the contrary. The concerns for meeting the aims and objective of the NHS business have appeared to supersede the internal professionalising agendas of an increasingly defensive and fragile nursing workforce. Some nurses have given up the fight and have left the NHS and nursing altogether, seeking a future in a new and more comfortable work environment (Mills 1998). Having said that, the picture so depressingly painted by Mills has clearly not applied to the whole of the nursing profession.

Thomas (1983) believed that nursing was standing up well to a government that was not committed to nurse professionalisation. He noted how the impact of a management-led organisation, significant education reform, a demographic decline and difficulties in recruiting staff were all pressing down on an increasingly beleaguered profession suffering from the developing reforms. That said, nurses had not just been reactive recipients to either those changes he noted, or indeed to the ones which have followed. Many have sought to strengthen, develop and change nursing's professional rationale, as society also has changed in its structure, and thus created new health needs to be met. Hart (1991), for example, reflected on nursing's ability to respond positively to the changes and challenges they have faced over time, both internally to their professional status within the health care service, and from wider external forces. It has often been difficult to prove the value of the professional nurse caring role to manager and policy maker alike. That said, these fundamental difficulties have provided the impetus for the pursuit and achievement of important theoretical developments in the understanding of the nature of nursing care, and these in turn have underpinned the creation of new practice. In a sense this hard travail of recent decades in pursuit of evidence to refute the notion that 'anyone can nurse', has prepared many within the profession well for the challenges and opportunities now offered by the present Government's proposed reforms (Cmd 3807 1997). However, before considering the future of the nursing profession under this Government, we will remind ourselves of just some of the agendas for professionalism which have been pursued, and which now underpin the nature of nurse care today.

AGENDA FOR NURSE PROFESSIONALISM

A major influence has been the introduction and development of the concept of 'new nursing' (Salvage 1988, 1990). This has shifted and changed both the philosophy and process of professional nurse care in practice, and has underpinned the Project 2000 reforms in nurse education. (United Kingdom Central Council 1986). According to Beardshaw & Robinson (1990), the changes implicit within this have involved 'moves to replace the task-based method of organising nursing work, with care more precisely tailored to individual patient needs'. In doing so, it sought 'to substitute a professional model of organisation for nursing's long established hierarchical, bureaucratic one'. Butterworth (1992) and Williams (1993) have seen these developments as a challenge to the biomedical ties of nursing to medicine, and as a recognition of the importance of the emotional and wider social aspects of care, health and well-being to the domains of nursing practice. In very practical terms, 'new nursing' emphasises a number of key issues:

◆ Nurse and client are active partners in care decisions and delivery.
◆ The nurse as educator has a goal of client empowerment.
◆ The client is the central focus of care – not the task.
◆ Care is specific and individualised to meet the needs of the client.
◆ An understanding of the broad determinants of health, and the holistic nature of client need, necessitates an exploration of the physical, intellectual, emotional, social and spiritual needs of individuals, community and society.
◆ The client is seen as an individual in a broad social context (family, community, society), and this will influence and impact both positively and negatively on the health and well-being, response to illness, and recovery of that individual at any one time.
◆ The delivery of effective nursing care relies upon collaboration with other carers, both formal and informal, the client and other potential users of the health services.

In general, the 'new nursing' approach has helped to make and keep professional nurse care relevant to the needs of the developing health care systems within society. At the same time it has provided the focus, enthusiasm and support both for new practice developments (United Kingdom Central Council 1986, Agnew 1995, Jowett 1997, Redfern 1997) and allied educational courses, both at pre- and post-qualification levels (Thomson 1998). Initiatives of interest include primary nursing, nursing beds, nurse development units, named nurse concept, nurse practitioners and consultants, a developing focus on specialist and advanced practice, and clinical management – to mention just a few.

So, in spite of the already noted 'inhospitable terrain', nurses have pursued professional status by a number of means. Notwithstanding these efforts, Salter & Snee (1997) believe that nursing's pursuit of professional status has been largely unsuccessful during this period. Others however refer positively to the many nurse-led developments that have been acknowledged and as such legitimised by mentions in government documents (NHSME 1993a, b). The present Government's new health agenda (Command 3807 1997) has also continued this apparent support for innovative professional nurse development.

However, it is clear that any future nurse professional developments will depend upon how much real support nurses are given by the government of the day and thus by health service management. During the internal market health reforms for example, there were many mixed messages being given to nurses relating to both professional survival, or indeed demise. Emphasis was often placed on the value of the whole nursing profession to the future of the NHS and to the provision of high quality health promoting care (Bottomley 1993). At the same time, support and interest clearly developed in the idea of skill mixing (Lightfoot, Baldwin & Wright 1992) and in the substitution of the financially costly nursing profession by a generic carer workforce (Manchester University 1996).

This latter proposal envisaged a health care workforce made up of an appropriately planned mix of differently skilled carers, remunerated according to skill level achieved, and employed because of their appropriateness to the needs of the care situation at any one time. Such flexibility of employment with the ability to skill-mix and thus to contain costs, clearly held appeal – not least to those who view nurse professionals as inappropriate and expensive rigidities within the health care employment market.

In many respects, the discussions around the need for skill-mixing, flexibility of working, and the fairness of payment linked to skills delivered, very much mirrors the arguments made on the ambulance workers' pay in the early 1980s. It was said then that as the skill levels involved varied from employee to employee, i.e broadly from taxi driver to paramedic, there was no reason to pay and reward the whole ambulance workforce at the same levels. Those who delivered at a high level of skill/knowledge, i.e. the highly skilled paramedic, deserved his title and financial reward commensurate with his contribution to health care delivery. Those, however, who transported clients to and from health care settings should be rewarded for their taxi service role, and be given a lower status than their more able colleagues. Similarly, then, within the nursing profession there have been moves to differentiate out role, task and financial reward, not least through the nurse grading system and the development of skill-mixing in care teams. In a sense, these moves have effectively divided up and emphasised different levels of skill and knowledge across the whole of the professional nurse workforce.

Over time, these sorts of moves have set apart and highlighted the well skilled and higher status, elite minority group of nurses, whether at practitioner, manager or academic levels. By contrast, their lesser skilled and lesser status majority counterparts have been similarly earmarked. However, as we have already seen, they have been strongly challenged as to the claimed professional status of their role and tasks.

Presently, the relatively recent Manchester Health Services Management Unit (HSMU) proposals for the development of a generic carer role are still on the table (Manchester University 1996). It clearly remains to be seen whether the new Government decides to revisit this particular legacy of Conservative health reforms.

That said, this is not an attempt to instil fear into nurse colleagues, but an expression of genuine concern. After all, qualified nursing care continues to remain a costly resource in the NHS budgeting equation, under whichever government. Because of this, no matter how well the profession redefines its roles, nursing, as in any other part of the labour market, will continue to be under close scrutiny, and subject to vigorous questioning as to its value and special status within the health care setting. As the Manchester University Report reminded us all:

> *The NHS employment culture has changed. In place of the old deal (loyalty, compliance and expertise, in exchange for regular promotion, salary increases and care in time of trouble), organisations now offer constant challenge, and they reward employees who are eager to meet it. In exchange, they expect flexibility, responsibility, accountability and the longest hours in Europe.*

So, what other skeletons might be still lying around to frighten the profession in the future?

WHISTLEBLOWING

The need to meet service requirements in the internal market in the most cost-effective way has certainly provided an often difficult backcloth to nurse professional development. Issues concerning autonomy of practice, pay commensurate with skills and knowledge and with comparable occupations, credibility of the nurse role and support for new developments in caring have all been under threat. The nursing press has been full of worrying individual and group experiences of the reforms, among many other things, relating to standards of care and to professional developments. A brief look at the whistleblowing issues will help to highlight some of the problems that have been felt by nurses during the past two decades.

Only a month after the implementation of the reforms in 1991, press reports described NHS management as beginning a process of restricting NHS staff from speaking out against the changes (Editorial 1991). Calls to restore the medical and nursing professionals' right to free speech without confidentiality clauses in contracts were widely discussed and reported. According to Waterhouse (1991):

> *Doctors, nurses and hospital staff who speak out against the Government's NHS reforms – in particular its plans for hospitals to become self-governing trusts – are being threatened with dismissal. Since the NHS reforms came into effect on 1st April, some authorities have imposed new "confidentiality" clauses in contracts without debate, in what the Royal College of Nursing describes as a "climate of intimidation".*

Almost inevitably examples have occurred of cases of individuals who in expressing their concerns about aspects of NHS standards or practice have found themselves subject to disciplinary procedures:

◆ Graham Pink described his concerns about the lack of staff on wards for elderly people in Stepping Hill Hospital, Stockport (Bolger 1990, Brindle 1990).

◆ Dr Helen Zeitlin spoke out against nursing shortages at Alexandra Hospital, Redditch, and was dismissed on grounds of redundancy (Snell 1992).

◆ Dr Chris Chapman (Biochemist, Leeds General Infirmary Trust) was sacked after he had unearthed a scientific fraud and went public. He was given notice after the reorganisation of the pathology department at LGI and was the only member of the 200 strong department to lose his job (Hugill 1992).

Not so well reported or known about was the threat by St Bartholomew's College of Nursing to discipline 22 third year students who had complained about standards of care in two clinical placements (Nursing Times 1992). The threat was removed after they had apologised for the offence they had caused by their letter. Incidentally, their complaints were acted upon, which suggests they were probably right in the first place. One could argue that this particular experience may well have ensured that some of them will keep their thoughts to themselves in the future – hardly helpful in encouraging them to apply their code of conduct (their badge of professional 'integrity') in future times, when another bad care experience faces them. Rundell, however, suggests that some nurses would actually prefer a full-blown gagging clause in their contract because this would avoid the obvious unpleasantness surrounding speaking out (Rundell 1992). As Wright explained:

> *The history of nursing is littered with the names of those lost to the profession who were unable to pursue and sustain a complaint. People like Mr Pink who hit the headlines are in the minority; thousands more are unable or unwilling to follow this path. (Wright 1990)*

Indeed, according to an MSF (Manufacturing, Science and Finance) union survey:

Nurses are less likely to "whistleblow" about standards of care than any other group of NHS employees – nurses were the most "vulnerable" and were afraid to speak out because they had neither the independent status of GPs nor the seniority of consultants. (MSF 1993)

This is a sad conclusion because nurses clearly have had concerns about the NHS. An RCN survey for example (Brindle 1993a) which questioned 2000 nurses found:

◆ Almost two in three nurses believed that there were too few staff on their wards to provide proper patient care.
◆ Only one in five nurses was confident that managers would act on concerns about staffing.

In a sense here we see the dilemma for nurses. They have clearly known the issues which should be raised, but they have been either frightened, or have felt that there was little use in speaking out. Indeed, if they have known anything about those who have hit the headlines and lost their jobs in the process, it is little wonder that they have kept quiet. As Derek Fatchett MP said at the launch of the pressure group 'Freedom to Care': 'Nurses and doctors who tell the truth about care in the NHS risk the sack' (Fatchett 1992). Could we really have confidence in Duncan Nichol's words on launching the previous Government's guidelines on whistleblowing? (NHSME 1993c). He said that 'it was important to encourage openness and dialogue in the NHS where the free expression by staff of their concerns were welcomed by their managers as a contribution towards improving services' (Snell 1993). Responses to the document included it being described as a 'gagger's charter' and 'creating a climate of fear' and a 'press gag on health staff' (Brindle 1993b).

Many commentators have referred to the dissonance between the previous government's expressed wishes, and the action taken on their behalf in the NHS. Nichols asserted that the NHS existed to meet the needs of patients, and affirmed the duty of all employees to draw to the attention of their managers any matter they considered to be damaging the interests of patients and clients. That is all very well, but according to one editor, the guidance did not deal with the possible disputes over large policy issues such as funding and staffing levels. There was no room for the nurse who spoke out because he felt the quality of patient care was being adversely affected by government policy. (Editorial 1993).

The fear of speaking out has sadly continued. According to Fursland (1996), despite fewer explicit clauses prohibiting employees from whistleblowing, the culture of secrecy in the NHS is alive and thriving. As she reported:

> *Although there may be fewer explicit gagging clauses in the NHS trust contracts than four years ago, the culture of secrecy is as strong as ever. Rather than blowing the whistle, people are nervous. They keep quiet, even though things are worrying them. Jobs are so insecure that they are afraid of stepping out of line and criticising management.*

Gulland (1997) also noted that it was still difficult for nurses to whistleblow because they risk retribution. They risked their jobs if they raised concerns, but breached their professional code of conduct if they did not. If this is the case, then so much for the value of the Nurse Code of Conduct (United Kingdom Central Council 1992). It would seem that in this particular respect, any claims to professional autonomy remain very much open to question. While there are those who remind us that there has always been in the lineage of nursing a tradition of compliance (Rowden 1992), we need to view the moves in recent years to quieten any potential dissenting professional nursing voice as something quite different in character.

In conclusion to this section, it is pleasing to note that the Conservative MP Richard Shepherd is presently putting a Public Interest Disclosure Bill through Parliament, apparently with the support of the Government. Its aim is to protect employees who raise concerns about malpractice, involving fraud, abuse in care, danger to public safety, damage to the environment and other wrongdoings.

As he has acknowledged:

> *Whatever the rights and wrongs of the NHS reforms, one of the most damaging side-effects has been the perception that NHS staff are too frightened to raise their concerns about patient care or financial malpractice and those that do speak up are gagged and victimised. (Shepherd 1998)*

It is to be hoped that in the near future whistleblowers will receive protection under employment law. If that is to be the case, nurses who do have concerns about patient care should feel more able to speak out and to demonstrate that their Code of Conduct is indeed a 'guarantee of professional integrity' (Kaye 1965).

PAY, CASUALISATION AND SKILL-MIXING

It would appear that nursing's many professionalising strategies during the last two decades seem to have been under constant challenge in one way or another. Any progress that has been achieved has clearly involved a good degree of individual tenacity and strength of purpose. The environment has not been favourable to the professionally faint hearted and the reasons are easy to discover.

First, nurses appear to have been increasingly controlled in what they say, and how they work. Second, successive derisory pay awards have suggested anything but professional credibility. The reality is that nursing as a group is expected to deliver each government's vision for health care, but in return the credibility being sought as 'full' professionals remains an apparently illusory objective for the majority of nurses.

Seccombe & Smith (1996) in their research on the nursing workforce found that 'for a growing proportion of nurses, particularly those in the NHS, there is a significant mismatch between the rewards, including pay, career prospects and working hours, offered by the work environment, and their needs and expectations'. Increasing workloads, the excessive hours of expected work, the need to do bank work as well as a main job, short term contracts, casualisation, shortages and cutbacks in equipment, – all have contributed to low professional morale. Naish in early 1997 referred to the findings of Nursing Times/ICM poll on the state of the profession. Sixty-seven per cent of the respondents said morale was either low or very low among their nursing colleagues. By the end of 1997, Unison's independently commissioned research as part of its 1998 evidence considered leaving the NHS or quitting the profession altogether (Payne 1997).

An editorial in 'Nursing Times' noted that in spite of these worrying trends: 'that workloads had snowballed as demands soared and technology became ever more complex. The staff who now remained were expected to do more with less, and whilst they had coped admirably to date, it was felt that they cannot, nor should not, carry on being exploited' (Editorial 1997) – clearly a hard message aimed at the Government.

THE FUTURE FOR PROFESSIONAL NURSING

So far this discussion has considered a variety of issues around the nature of professionalism, with specific emphasis on nursing. The backcloth to the many points raised has been that of the NHS internal market reforms, which as we know from previous chapters appear to have produced dissonance between, on the one hand, the public statements of support for enhanced nurse professionalism, and on the other, the actual pressures upon the nurse role. It is this dissonance which inevitably has caused some concern for the future of nursing as a profession. The question therefore now has to be, can the difficult tide of recent years be turned?

Initial responses to this may be surprisingly upbeat. After all, the many perceived and real barriers to professional development have singularly failed to halt the creation of innovative and relevant nurse responses to the ever-challenging health needs agenda. New skills have been developed in order to improve the standard of care offered. These have, for example, included research and evidence-based practice, quality and standard setting, audit, assessment of health need, health promotion and education, the creation of care protocols, the evaluation of care and multidisciplinary collaboration. In a sense then, while the roughness of the reforms may well have proved just too much for many nurses, others have not only survived, but developed as professionals. They are now even better equipped to tackle the future in the new primary care-led NHS. For many, the promised developments in the NHS offer at long last an important way forward for professional nursing. The proposals are seen as recognising the value and expertise of its contribution. As Hancock points out:

Nurse involvement in the new NHS has been given a big emphasis. The government is particularly keen to extend what it describes as the recent development in the roles of nurses working in acute and community services. (Hancock 1998)

Baroness Jay (Health Minister responsible for nursing) has made it clear that the Government recognises the critical contribution of nurses to the achievement of a modern and effective NHS (Jay 1997). She has set out a number of initiatives to be taken up by nurses, which not only reflect the importance given to the profession, but will surely help to raise its profile in the future. The initiatives proposed are:

◆ Nurse-led 24-hour national help and advice line (NHS Direct).
◆ Leadership roles on primary care groups.
◆ National task force, including nurses, to identify good practice.
◆ Quality and standard setting – locally and regionally.
◆ Creation of clinical guidelines on clinical cost effectiveness (National Institute for Clinical Excellence).
◆ New commission for health improvement to support and oversee the quality of clinical services.

The Chief Nursing Officer is also to begin work on the development of a new strategy for nursing, midwifery and health visiting. According to Jay (1997), this is to allow nurses to take on wider professional responsibilities, as well as to build on the core of present nursing practice.

In conclusion, there appear to be opportunities opening up within the NHS for those nurses who have the professional skills and willingness to rise to the challenges being offered by the Government (Fatchett 1998). Having said that, we need to look back at Asvall's statements at the beginning of the chapter. While he has no doubt as to the importance of nursing's professional contributions to society, he reminds us that society and governments also have a duty to provide nurses with the recognition they deserve, and the working conditions they need to carry out their unique role. The future for professional nursing rests not just within itself, but in a reciprocal partnership with the whole of the community.

REFERENCES

Ackroyd S 1992 In: Soothill K, Henry C, Kendrick K (eds) Themes in nursing. Chapman and Hall, London, ch 19

Agnew T 1995 A change of part. Nursing Times 91(43): 20–21

Allsop J 1995 Health, policy and the NHS: towards 2000, 2nd edn. Longman, London

Asvall JE 1997 In: Salvage J, Heijnen S (eds) Nursing in Europe. A better resource for health. WHO regional publications. European Series No 74. WHO, Geneva

Beardshaw V, Robinson R 1990 New for old? Prospects for nursing in the 1990s. No 8 Research Report Series Current Health Policy Issues. Kings Fund, London

Becker H S 1970 Sociological work.Allen Lane, London

Benzeval M, Judge K, Whitehead M 1995 Tackling inequalities in health. Kings Fund, London

Bolger T 1990 Can you hear the whistle? Nursing Times, 86(18): 18, 24

Bottomley V 1993 In: NHSME. A vision for the future. Department of Health, London pii

Bridges J 1991 Distinct from medicine. Nursing Times 87(27): 42–43

Brindle D 1990 Yours sincerely, F.G. Pink. The Guardian, 11 April

Brindle D 1993a Nurses say too few staff for proper patient care. The Guardian, 17 May

Brindle D 1993b Press 'gag' on health staff. The Guardian, 10 June

Brindle D 1993c Doctors, nurses . . . and managers. (Health appointments) The Guardian, 29 September p 15

Brown J 1996 Robot nurses nonsense. Nursing Standard 10(47): 10

Butterworth T 1992 Clinical supervision as an emerging idea in nursing. In: Butterworth T, Faugier J (eds) Clinical supervision and mentorship in nursing. Chapman and Hall, London

Caines E 1996 Goodbye nurses. Nursing Standard 10(39): 18

Chapman P 1996 In: Agnew T. Generic carers should replace nurses, says report. Nursing Times 92(21): 5

Cohen P 1993 United fronts? Nursing Times 89(26): 40–41

Command 555 1989 Working For Patients. HMSO, London

Command 3807 1997 The New NHS. Modern. Dependable. HMSO, London

Conroy M 1996 In: Leifer D. Designing new workers for tomorrow's world. Nursing Standard 10(36): 14

Davies C 1995 Gender and the professional predicament in nursing. Open University Press, Milton Keynes

Davies C 1996a Cloaked in a tattered illusion. Nursing Times 92(45): 44–46

Davies C 1996b A new vision of professionalism. Nursing Times 92(46): 54–56

Donaldson L 1995 The Listening Blank. Health Service Journal, 25 September 25, pp. 22–24

Durkheim E 1951 Suicide: a study in sociology. Free Press, New York

Dyson 1993 In: Downey R. Call for freeze on student intakes. Nursing Times 89(14): 6

Editorial 1991 Stealthy is not very healthy. The Guardian, 20 May

Editorial 1993 A charter with no teeth. Nursing Times, 89(24): 5

Editorial 1996 Cloak of professionalism. Nursing Times 92(45): 3

Editorial 1997 Comment. Nursing Times 93(43): 3

English T 1996 In: Healey P. President of BMA condemns idea of generic workforce as 'nonsense'. Nursing Standard 10(39): 7

Etzioni A 1969 The semi-professions and their organisation: teachers, nurses, social workers. Free Press, New York

Exworthy M 1996 Power points. Health Service Journal 106(5504): 24–25

Fatchett A 1996 A chance for community nurses to shape the health agenda. Nursing Times 92(45): 40–42

Fatchett A 1998 Where next? The Yorkshire Practice Nurse Association Journal. Winter, pp 3–4

Fatchett D 1992 Government guidance on free speech given cool response. Nursing Times 88(47): 6

Faugier J 1992 Tall Poppies. Nursing Times 88(50): 20

Friedson E 1970 The profession of medicine. Dodd Mead, London

Fursland E 1996 Still gagging on the truth. The Guardian, 20 November, p 9

Gamarnikow E 1978 Sexual division of labour: the case in nursing. In: Kuhn A, Wolpe A (eds) Feminism and materialism. Routledge and Kegan Paul, London

Game A, Pringle R 1983 Gender at work. Pluto Press, London

Gillan J 1994 The cull. Nursing Times 90(3): 56

Goodchild G 1995 The Jack of all trades is master of none. Nursing Times 92(24): 24

Gough P 1997 Time to grasp the nettle. Nursing Times 93(12): 26–27

Greenwood E 1957 Attributes of a profession. Social Work 2(3): 44–45

Griffiths R 1983 NHS Management Inquiry. Department of Health, London

Gulland A 1997 Inquiry calls for formal help for whistleblowers. Nursing Times 93(9): 10

Haggard S 1995 In: Tomlin Z. Blame the system. Health Service Journal June, p. 12

Hancock C 1996 With the benefit of foresight. Health Service Journal 27 June, p. 23

Hancock C 1998 Party to the vision of the future. Health Service Journal 15 January, p 20

Hansard Parliamentary Debates 1989 Statement. NHS Review 146(39): 165–189

Hart E 1991 Ghost in the machine. Health Service Journal 5 December, pp 20–22

Heller T 1978 Restructuring the health service. Croom Helm, London

Holliday I 1992 The NHS Transformed. Baseline Books, Manchester

Hugill B 1992 Fraud probe after hospital sacks its whistle-blower. The Observer, 11 October

Hugman R 1991 Power in caring professions. Macmillan, Basingstoke

Jay M 1997 The White Paper recognises that nurses have a critical contribution to make. Nursing Times 93(51): 3

Johnson TJ 1972 Professions and power. Macmillan, London

Jowett S 1997 The impact of scope. Nursing Times 93(52):

Kaye B 1965 In: Prandy K. Professional employees. Faber and Faber, London

Kenny C 1997a Leaflets to replace nurses. Nursing Times 93(25): 8

Kenny C 1997b Nurses the key to health savings. Nursing Times 93(34): 7

Kenny C 1997 Trust defies minister's call to stop cutting jobs. Nursing Times 93(49): 6

Liefer D 1996 Designing new workers for tomorrow's world. Nursing Standard 10(36): 14

Lightfoot J, Baldwin S, Wright K 1992 Nursing by numbers? Setting staffing levels for district nursing and health visiting services. Social Policy Research Unit, University of York, York

Manchester University 1996 The future health care workforce. Health Service Management Unit (HSMU), Manchester

Mangan P 1993 Survival of the fittest. Nursing Times 89(6): 26

McEvoy P 1992 The professionals. Nursing Times 88(9): 40–41

Meehan F 1996 A lesson learned (Editorial). Journal of Community Nursing 10(9):

Mihill C 1996 GP exodus threatens NHS disaster. The Guardian, 26 June, p 8

Millerson G 1964 The qualifying associations: a study in professionalism. Routledge and Kegan Paul, London

Mills B 1998 Degree of sacrifice. The Guardian (Society) 21 January, pp 2–3

MSF (Manufacturing, Science and Finance Union) 1993 Nursing staff too afraid to speak out on standards of care. Nursing Times 89(9)

Murray T 1990 The college's response to the ambulance dispute does not reflect credit on nursing. Nursing Times, 86(7): (letters)

Naish J 1997 Future shock. Nursing Times 93(6): 34–36

NHSME (National Health Service Management Executive) 1993a New world. New opportunities. Department of Health, London

NHSME (National Health Service Management Executive) 1993b A Vision for the Future. Department of Health, London

NHSME (National Health Service Management Executive) 1993c Guidance for staff on relations with the public and the media. Department of Health, London

Nightingale F 1881 Letter to probationer nurses at St Thomas's Hospital. In: Nightingale Collection LSE

Nocon A 1994 Collaboration in community care in the 1990's. Business Education Publishers, Sunderland, Tyne and Wear

North N, Bradshaw Y 1997 Perspectives in health care. Macmillan, Basingstoke

Nursing Times 1992 College drops actions as students apologise 88(41): 8

Nursing Times 1996 Pandora's box of tricks. Nursing Times 92(15): 3

Oakley A 1984 What price professionalism? The importance of being a nurse. Nursing Times 7: 24–27

Parsons T 1939 The professions and the social structure. Social Forces 17: 457–467

Parsons T 1951 The social system, Routledge and Kegan Paul, London

Payne D 1997 Unison warns of nurse exodus. Nursing Times 93(42): 5

Peters BD 1978 In: Lewis PG, Potter DC, Castles FG (eds) The practice of comparative politics. Longman, London

Pilkington E 1989 Angels with battered wings. The Guardian 29 November

Redfern S 1997 Reactions to nurses' expanding practice. Nursing Times 93(32): 45–47

Robinson J 1991 Power, politics and policy analysis in nursing. In: Perry A, Jolley M (eds) Nursing: a knowledge base for practice. Edward Arnold, London

Rowden R 1992 Self-imposed silence. Nursing Times 88(24): 31

Rundell S 1991 Who wants to be a doctor? Nursing times 87(1): 12

Rundell S 1992 Bound up. Nursing Times 88(37): 24

Salter B, Snee N 1997 Power dressing. Health Service Journal, 13 February

Salvage J 1988 Professionalisation – or struggle for survival? Journal of Advanced Nursing 13: 515–519

Salvage J 1990 The theory and practice of the new nursing. Nursing Times 86(4): 42–45

Seccombe I, Smith G 1996 Voting with their feet. Nursing Standard 11(1): 22–23

Shelley H 1993 Why tall poppies are not popular. Nursing Times 89(4): 12

Shepherd R 1998 In: Butler P. Wetting the whistle. Health Service Journal 29 January, p. 12

Snell J 1992 Whistle-blowing doctor to get job back. Nursing Times 88(46) 9

Snell Janet 1993b Whistleblower guide comes under attack. Nursing Times 89(24): 7

Spurgeon P 1997 How nurses can influence policy. Nursing Times 93(45): 34–35

Thomas B 1993 A dilution of skills. Nursing Times 89(29): 30–31

Thomson S 1998 After Project 2000: what does the future hold for nursing education? Nursing Times 94(3): 60–61

Thornton C 1995 In: Cain P, Hyde V, Hawkins E. Community nursing. Dimensions and Dilemmas. Arnold, London, pp 110–143

Turner BS 1991 Medical power and social knowledge. Sage, London

United Kingdom Central Council 1986 Project 2000: a new preparation for practice. UKCC, London

United Kingdom Central Council 1992 Code of professional conduct for the nurse, midwife and health visitor, 3rd edn. UKCC, London

Waterhouse R 1991 NHS staff gagged on health reforms. Independent on Sunday, 12 May

Watkins SJ 1992 The trouble with nursing. Health Visitor 65(10):

Weber M 1966 The sociology of religion. Methuen, London

Williams J 1993 What is a profession? Experience versus expertise. In: Beattie A, Gott M, Jones L, Sidell M (eds) Health and well-being: a reader. Macmillan Open University, Basingstoke

Witts P 1992 In: Soothill K, Henry C and Kendrick K (eds) Themes and perspectives in nursing. Chapman and Hall, London, pp 158–180

Wright S 1990 How the nurses can gain the power to speak out. The Guardian 25 August

Collaborative care

*Modern health care relies increasingly on team work; the development of
multi-professional teams, working not only in hospital and primary care
settings, but across the traditional boundaries of health and social care.
(Cmd 3425 1996)*

The promotion of the concept of collaboration has been, and remains, an
important theme underpinning current health policy activity. It is succinctly
defined by Øvretveit, Mathias & Thompson (1993) as:

Organisations or individuals working together or acting jointly.

The development of its application in practice across diverse health and
social care fields has been widely researched and analysed (Leathard 1994,
Øvretveit, Mathias & Thompson 1997), and reasons given for the apparent
surge in popularity for collaboration include:

◆ A growth in the complexity of health and welfare services.
◆ Expansion of knowledge and subsequent increase in specialisation
  (Marshall et al 1979).
◆ A perceived need for the rationalisation of resources.
◆ A need for lessening the duplication of care.
◆ The provision of a more effective, integrated and supportive service for
  both users and professionals.

The health and social care policies implicit within the NHS and
Community Care Act (1990) embodied all of the reasons given above. The Act
created a planning framework in which agencies had to work much more
closely together, and placed great emphasis on consultation and collaboration
at every level (Audit Commission 1992). This has not been easy to achieve.
During recent years, health and social carers have faced a difficult dilemma
as they have tried to implement policies, the focus of which has often seemed
implicitly to be in conflict. On the one hand there have been exhortations to
collaborate, and to provide eclectic and appropriately broad responses to
health need. On the other hand, the formation of the internal health care
market has fostered an environment of competition and secrecy between

carers and providers – an environment not necessarily conductive to multi-agency collaboration.

According to the analysis of Flynn, Williams & Pickard (1997):

Co-ordination has been made more difficult with the change, variety and complexity of health and social services in the 1990's.

However, the previous Conservative health administration appeared not to see any such problems. They set out their interpretation in the following way:

We need constructive co-operation between different parts of the NHS as well as the beneficial impact of competition. Improving health care is not a question of balancing one or the other. We have to find the appropriate balance between the two. (NHSME 1994)

The achievement of 'the appropriate balance' has not been easily secured in the NHS. Nocon (1994), in his work on calls for better collaboration, noted little positive impact, not least because 'the process (collaboration) is a difficult one, the rewards uncertain, and organisations often have (had) other priorities'. The internal market reforms in effect have made collaboration more difficult both within and without the NHS organisation.

This chapter will consider a number of issues which are pertinent to this discussion, and which may elucidate and develop some of the points already made. These will include:

1. Commercialisation and collaboration.
2. The NHS reforms – the creation of a low trust environment.
3. The creation of low trust relationships – a theoretical model.
4. The creation of high trust relationships – collaborative potential?
5. The Labour Government's health care proposals – the need for effective collaboration.
6. Changes needed in structure and organisation.
7. Professional development and support.

COMMERCIALISATION AND COLLABORATION

In earlier chapters, it has been argued that the process of reform has added a new commercial dimension to the culture of the NHS. In turn, it is felt that this commercialisation has created a climate of great uncertainty, suspicion, confusion and low morale among many health care workers. (Fatchett 1996, Rillands 1997). These feelings have erected a barrier to effective collaborative ventures. Platt (1997), for instance, referred to the ongoing difficulty of getting people in the health service 'out of thinking about the market and competition, and thinking more of coherent planning and collaboration'.

It seems that for many the changes have not been conducive to the creation of professional care environments, underpinned by trusting and smooth working collaborative relationships between a wide range of professionals, organisations, users and carers. The internal health care market has created metaphorical demarcation lines between fragmented provider units. In turn, many health service employees have felt unable, or have indeed been forbidden to collaborate externally in any meaningful way. Commercial secrecy between competitor provider units bidding against each other for contracts has become a central theme (Best & Brazil 1997). Collaboration with other potential NHS competitors, and indeed with wider agencies, whatever the depth of their relationship previous to the reforms, appears to have taken a back seat in recent times. As Kurtz & Nicholl (1992) said:

Where there was collaboration, there is now invoicing; where there was give and take, there are now accountants bent on capturing "items of service".

Having said that, it would be unfair to blame a lack of multidisciplinary collaboration in care on organisational and structural changes alone. As Trevillion (1995) reminds us:

Collaboration is as much about an organisational culture as well as a practitioner culture.

While the increasingly commercialised and competitive environment in the NHS has no doubt sharpened up the organisational culture, in turn, the professionals within that context have contributed their own practitioner culture too. The fact should not be ignored that over time professional groups have perpetuated a 'Berlin wall of secrecy', a lack of willingness to collaborate with others; not only outside their own organisation, but sadly even within. Hugman (1995) refers to those who are 'inward-looking and too defensive of established practice' to work with others. While that may well have been true for many, Ross & Mackenzie (1996) offer a broader and more eclectic explanation for professional difficulties in collaboration:

It is perhaps a reflection of the complex conceptual, structural and professional issues that lie at its roots, that have resulted in slow progress of understanding, interpretation, and implementation in practice.

They note the many attempts to analyse the concept of collaboration, and in turn to offer constructive solutions for progress (Meek & Pietroni 1993, Leathard 1994, Nocon 1994, Poulton & West 1994, Owens & Carrier 1995, Flynn, Williams & Pickard 1997, Boarden 1997, Øvretveit, Mathias & Thompson 1997). The fact that the process has been examined from diverse theoretical perspectives, including psychology, sociology, social policy, economics, organisation and management, government and social administration, suggests that effective collaboration in care is not easily achieved, and that there are no easy answers either to the problems of ineffective collaboration. The process is exceedingly difficult to do well. While no doubt this observation is true, the almost in-built and historical professional antipathy towards multi-disciplinary collaboration has clearly not helped the situation to develop in as constructive and as positive manner as might have been possible during the period of reform.

It is not difficult to suggest a number of reasons why many individuals have metaphorically dug in their professional heels. The imposition of General Managers, with the apparent reduction in the importance attached to the professional voice, has led to the development of a low trust and very defensive approach to practice on the part of many professionals. From this position it is easy to see how such individuals may have felt unable to become the type of trusting people who might create a caring sharing relationship with others, and not least with those who are in a potential competitive relationship with them. The analysis by Flynn, Williams & Pickard of developing high and low trust relationships during the period of the NHS reforms, engendered by the new contracting culture, provides a helpful model to highlight and to explain professional responses, not least in relation to collaboration. As Flynn, Williams & Pickard conclude:

> *Central government instruction to promote contestability, accountability and value for money ultimately came to dominate their commissioning and contracting approach. The effect was too often to corrode rather than nurture common values and commitments, to create an atmosphere of mistrust and to exacerbate inherent problems of uncertainty in the contract process. (Flynn, Williams & Pickard 1997)*

In all fairness we may need to conclude at this stage that the blame for a lack of successful collaboration lies both with professionals themselves and with organisational structures. The reality is that a great deal of work and goodwill is needed to make successful collaboration happen. Understanding of its nature by both professional and policy maker alike needs to move beyond the easy and often stated acknowledgement that 'it is a good thing', and 'needs to take place if effective care services are to be provided'. According to Hudson (1997):

> *Although the centre can create a legal, administrative and financial framework that facilitates such collaboration, these are not characteristics that can be conjured up by administrative fiat. The real issue – whether at professional or organisational level – is whether or not there is a willingness to align decisions. And this is a question of politics, personalities and culture, rather than one of legislation and finance.*

Hudson's conclusion perhaps reflects the old saying: where there is a will, there is a way. That said, apparently insuperable organisational barriers to collaboration, as noted earlier, have confounded many in practice during the past years. Most practitioners believe like Nocon that:

Collaboration between health and social care agencies can help ensure that the totality of people's needs is both recognised and met. However, the fragmentation of organisations, and the creation of a health and social care divide (Cmd 555 1989, Cmd 849 1989), have hindered the good delivery of many important policy developments requiring multidisciplinary collaboration.

Discharge planning from hospital, 'The Health of the Nation' initiatives, cross-sector care of the mentally ill; the elderly; the disabled, and child protection work, for example, have often proved difficult to implement in a high quality collaborative manner.

Roberts & Priest (1997) have referred to the competitive character of contemporary service provision, with its conflicting policy perspectives, pay differentials, status and budgetary concerns (which have tended to perpetuate role separation), to inhibit effective collaboration, and to fragment the delivery of care. The alternative or more balanced solution to the continuing search for the holy grail of effective collaboration must then rely on:

1. The development of an organisational structure and culture which actively promotes working together rather than being in directly competitive relationships.

2. Greater professional understanding of, and enthusiasm for the concept and process of collaborative working.

An immediate question is: will this happen in the foreseeable future? A positive response at this stage would suggest a large degree of hope over experience. It becomes obvious that the Government's White Paper (Cmd 3807 1997) and its hoped for policy developments can only achieve success on implementation, if the collaborative principles underpinning them are addressed in equally serious measure also. The new ideas, professional and public support all need to be harnessed into a collective and collaborative effort and will. It is not sufficient to tell or to ask people to work together, or even to pretend that they are, when they are not. In turn, structures and organisations are needed in which people can work together and feel enabled to do so. That said, even if some serious and meaningful effort is put into the collaborative agenda by the Government, the trends and negative nuances of the previous years may well continue to have a stultifying effect on the multidisciplinary programme being proposed. However, before developing this line of discussion, we will consider how and why the NHS reforms of recent years appear to have created a low trust, anticollaborative environment. In turn, it should be possible to see how a high trust environment might be created in the future – one which will help the new reforms to be more successful than those of the previous Government.

THE NHS REFORMS – THE CREATION OF A LOW TRUST ENVIRONMENT

The impact of the health reforms, as we have seen already, was the creation of a very complex and often challenging environment for care, one which was not always conducive to effective collaboration. In many situations professional carers may well have felt too preoccupied with the ever-changing imperatives of their own employer agendas, to reach out and to work in partnership with others. The recurring waves of new and ever-developing trends have kept professionals metaphorically on their toes, and certainly unable to relax in any professional way throughout the whole period of reform. Trends of importance certainly include:

◆ A competitive and commercialised environment and a contract culture.
◆ Search for value for money, cost efficiency and effectiveness.
◆ Setting of quality standards.
◆ Audits of clinical effectiveness.
◆ More overt rationing.
◆ Promotion of research-based care.
◆ Rationalised/smaller acute sector, closures and mergers.
◆ Decrease in dependency upon inpatient beds.
◆ Shorter hospital inpatient stays, early discharge, increased throughput.
◆ Shift in resources from hospital to primary care settings.
◆ Transfer of care from hospital/institution to home/homely settings.
◆ Change in balance of power and focus for care from hospital to general practice – the primary care-led NHS.
◆ A positive health agenda and health promotion targets.
◆ A split in organisational health and social care agendas.
◆ An increasing interest in self-help and personal responsibility for health and social care.
◆ The empowerment of consumers.
◆ Promotion of care by informal carers and other neighbourhood networks.
◆ The promotion of multiagency collaboration with all sectors concerned with care to collaborate in both planning and implementation.

According to the Conservative Government in 1996 (Cmd 3425 1996), there were many positive outcomes as a result of the introduction of their health reforms. The Government referred to an improvement in the overall health of the nation. In addition, they pointed out that the provision of services had remained available to all, on the basis of need, regardless of the ability to pay. Treatment and care had been targeted to meet local needs, with a continuous improvement in the quality of care provided. They also praised the efficient use of resources in meeting public expectations and demands. This positive resume is of little surprise. No government of any political persuasion has described their policy progress in negative terms, and certainly not in the run up to a general election.

The Conservatives' intentions, had they won the election of 1997, was to build on the structures they had put in place and to develop the services which the NHS offered its patients (Cmd 3425 1996). Collaboration and cooperation across all sectors were to have remained as important themes underpinning all future developments. As the then Secretary of State, Dorrell stated:

The delivery of health objectives requires the NHS to work closely with other agencies, both voluntary and statutory. In particular, it will only be possible to secure the fullest benefit from NHS resources against the background of close co-operation with social services. (Command 3425 1996)

This positive statement in support of a continuing collaborative approach appeared, however, to gloss over the many real difficulties practitioners have faced in trying to fashion such an agenda in an environment apparently more intent on pursuing financial objectives. During the period of NHS reform collaboration was a much promoted but often secondary objective to the task of developing the internal health care market. As Ross & Mackenzie (1996) noted, conflicts arose 'when the motive to work interprofessionally' was more geared 'towards securing business and contracts', than in the pursuit of client interest.

Hunter (1997), in his analysis of the impact of the reforms on NHS personnel, offered several telling pointers to the apparent lack of effective, professionally led collaborative effort. He referred to the emergence of a number of controversial workforce issues, such as the fragmentation of care provision, short term employment contracts, casualisation and skill mixing. These have engendered individual feelings of employment instability and insecurity. The sharper commercialised environment and the quantitative nature of contracting, have eroded the qualitative niceties and subtleties of care, in favour of the more easily measurable. As a result the special and professional nature of nurse caring has been challenged on many occasions. Arguments have been made that nursing care can be, and is, carried out just as effectively, and certainly more cheaply, by non-professionals. The outcome of these developments has been the development of low trust relationships between many individuals – the very opposite of the reciprocal feelings needed to make effective collaborative care happen.

THE CREATION OF LOW-TRUST RELATIONSHIPS – A THEORETICAL MODEL

Flynn, Williams & Pickard's (1997) work on contracting in community health services provides a detailed and interesting critical commentary on how markets and networks have evolved in the purchaser–provider framework for community health services. Specifically for this discussion there is an analysis of workplace relationships, both high and low trust, engendered by the contracting process. Fox's work on authority, employment relationships and the degree of trust engendered in differing economic exchanges/ environments is used as a model for their analysis (Fox 1974).

Flynn, Williams & Pickard propose:

There is a complex dialectic of trust-distrust which affects all social relationships, but it is especially manifest in all forms of economic exchange and contractual behaviour.

We might consider this statement in relation to professional behaviour as the reforms of the NHS have developed in relation to both the introduction of general management and the internal health care market. As we have already noted, many professionals have become increasingly distrustful of others, whether colleague or manager, because of the professionally constraining environment created by the more bureaucratic and corporatist NHS agenda and style. The importance of competing for, winning, and holding contacts has encouraged a climate of enforced secrecy and confidentiality within individual provider units. Alongside this, professional voices and choices have been effectively stifled by increasingly powerful management executives. The apparently unfettered professional discretion which, according to Griffiths (1983), existed in the NHS previous to the introduction of general management, has come under tight financial and functional control. Professionals in a very general sense may well have concluded from their new relationships with powerful general managers that they are not trusted, and that their discretion and judgement around care activity have been effectively circumscribed and reduced in both content and flexibility. It is easy to see how the relationships between professionals and managers have turned and soured into one of low trust. In turn, with such feelings around, it is not difficult to see why collaboration in care has often been unsuccessful or indeed at times proved impossible.

Fox (1974) offers a theoretical explanation for this negative and potentially destructive situation. He found that if work activity is formalised and thus constrained, then the low trust relationship which is engendered between the worker and the authority figure will create a number of significant attitudes and attributes which make working together difficult.

Low trust relationships in work create participants who:

◆ Have divergent goals and interests.
◆ Have explicit expectations which must be reciprocated through balanced exchanges.
◆ Carefully calculate the costs and benefits of any concession made.
◆ Restrict and screen communications in their own separate interests.
◆ Attempt to minimise their dependence on other's discretion.
◆ Are suspicious about mistakes or failures, attributing them to ill-will or default, and invoke sanctions.

All or some of these aspects may reflect to some degree or other the reasons why many professional practitioners have not collaborated with others either seriously or effectively in the past years.

That said, personal, professional and structural barriers created by the reforms have in combination discouraged collaborative activity, or made it that more difficult. The commercialised and contractual nature of the NHS relationships both internally and outside of the organisation have seemingly replaced its altruistic nature (surely a necessary attribute for collaboration and interprofessional trust) with that of a cash nexus.

As Fox (1974) puts it:

The keen calculative specificity of reciprocation which characterises purely market transactions is a contradiction in terms to high discretion relations.

Local authority social carers, according to Hadley & Clough (1996), have also faced similar difficulties in their collaborative efforts. On the one hand they have felt the constraints of their own commercialised community care environment and, in addition, faced problems in collaborating across the fragmented and increasingly pluralised agencies on both sides of the health and social care divide (Johnston 1994). Without a doubt, the ever-increasing breadth and diversity of primary carers, all with differing aims and employer allegiances, have made joint working and shared responsibility nearly impossible at times.

Øvretveit (1993) appears to arrive at a similar conclusion. He finds that:

Neither market nor bureaucratic modes of organisation facilitate collaboration; co-ordination is more difficult to obtain where the actors' interests and issues are divergent, and where they have different objectives. Associational or network approaches are preferred as most likely to secure more effective co-ordination, but these are weakened by the impact of market competition.

Øvretveit thus looks to the creation of a more appropriate networking environment, one which requires and promotes a different set of relationships, which are not about competition or contractual strait jackets, but which emphasise trust, warmth, flexibility and sharing. Such attributes should encourage altruism and not self-interested individualism in care. In effect, there is a need to replace the low trust scenario to one of high trust, and to emphasise a belief in professionals' ability to make choices, to take risks and to use their discretion in meeting client need. It is perhaps in these circumstances, and with such relationships of trust, that collaborative efforts are more likely to take place, and potentially to meet with success.

THE CREATION OF HIGH-TRUST RELATIONSHIPS – COLLABORATIVE POTENTIAL?

We need to return briefly again to Fox's analysis (Fox 1974). He refers to the creation of high trust relationships in work. The attributes of such participants would suggest a perspective on life and work which is supportive of the sort of collaborative environment proposed by Øvretveit. High trust participants seem to exemplify the converse picture and package of attributes surrounding the low trust participants. For nurses, it is worth considering whether their own experiences at work and of colleague behaviour to one another during the period of reform matches up in any way to the positive description which follows.

High trust relationships in work create participants who:

◆ Share (or have similar) ends and values.
◆ Have a diffuse serve of long-term obligation.
◆ Offer support without calculating the cost or expecting an immediate return.
◆ Communicate freely and openly with one another.
◆ Are prepared to trust the other and risk their own fortunes in the other party.
◆ Give the benefit of the doubt in relation to motives and goodwill if there are problems.

Fox's perspectives on the creation of high and low trust relationships in the working environment thus offers a model of attributes and attitudes ranging through a continuum of low and high trust. In real life these ideal typical models, as portrayed by the opposing ends of the continuum, are not totally reflective of individuals' positions in practice. Individuals in reality will shift along the continuum depending on time, circumstance and need. As already suggested, the structure and organisation of the internal health care market have tended to push professionals and others towards the low trust end of the continuum. In the main, a tightened structure and corporate agenda have not been encouraging of flexible and collaborative ventures. At the same time, Trevillion's earlier comment on the effect of practitioner culture on collaborative effort should not be ignored (Trevillion 1995). While no doubt the old professional barriers have still come into play, the pursuit of economic aims and objectives has not necessarily harnessed the collective will and enthusiasm of professional participants. As such, it has created a low trust competitive environment in which multidisciplinary collaboration has been very much a secondary agenda. As noted before, Platt (1997) comments about NHS personnel from the perspective of a social services employee. She refers to them as now being stuck in an internalised mind-set of short term competition, and as such almost unable to think about long term planning and collaboration in care. Smith et al (1993) and Wistow (1992), for example, noted the lacklustre degree of collaboration by professionals with the voluntary sector – an observation which was not new (NCVO 1986). And, while ventures between the statutory sector and voluntary groups had been described as limited, bland and non-committal, efforts made to work with users and their informal carers were even less propitious. The centrality and value of their contribution to the success of health and social care delivery were barely recognised, and their views were often ignored in the process of care planning. Sadly, then, the long erected professional barriers to multidisciplinary working have been consolidated and continue to be maintained. It would seem that this attitude of disinterest in working together is persisting, whether caused by structure or organisation, or indeed because of professional antipathy. As such the future does not necessarily bode well for the successful delivery of the new health policy developments being introduced by the Government.

THE LABOUR GOVERNMENT'S HEALTH CARE PROPOSALS: THE NEED FOR EFFECTIVE COLLABORATION

This White Paper marks a turning point for the NHS. It replaces the internal market with integrated care. We are saving £1 billion of red tape and putting the money into front-line patient care. For the first time the need to ensure that high quality care is spread throughout the service will be taken seriously. National standards of care will be guaranteed. There will be easier and swifter access to the NHS when you need it. Our approach combines efficiency and quality with a belief in fairness and partnership. (Foreword by the Prime Minister Tony Blair (Cmd 3807 1997))

The concept of collaboration is one of the six key underpinning principles which underlies all of the changes proposed in the White Paper. As it clearly states:

*If these are to be a success, then there is a need for the NHS to work in
partnership, to break down organisational barriers, to forge stronger links
with Local Authorities, and to put the needs of the patient at the centre of
the care process. (2.4)*

A number of proposals for action and change in the NHS, both within this
document, and indeed in the February Green Paper on health (Cmd 3852
1998), can only hope to work if collaboration in care is pursued with some
seriousness by all participants – the public, the professionals and the politicians. The notion of partnership is thus broad and all inclusive. Rather than
health professionals 'doing' and 'deciding' for others within care relationships,
the onus now is on reciprocal partnerships and responsibilities. These will be
approached in a number of ways.

The important aim of reducing health inequalities, for example, will
require collaboration:

*The Government will ensure the NHS works locally with those who provide
social care, housing, education and employment, just as the Government
itself will work nationally across Whitehall to bring about lasting
improvements in the public's health. (1.2)*

The negative impacts of the internal market reforms on collaborative care
potential will be removed:

*The introduction of the internal market by the previous Government
prevented the health service from properly focusing on the needs of patients.
It wasted resources administering competition between hospitals. This White
Paper sets out how the internal market will be replaced by a system we have
called "integrated care" based on partnership and driven by performance.
(1.3)*

The fragmenting impact of the internal market reforms on planning, funding and delivering of health care will be removed. It had provided little strategic coordination and had been poorly placed to tackle the crucial issue of
better integration between health and social care. To overcome this, a new
collaborative mechanism would be introduced, that of the Health
Improvement Programme' (HIP).

*In the New NHS all those charged with planning and providing health and
social care services for patients will work to a jointly agreed local Health
Improvement Programme. This will govern the actions of all parts of the
local NHS to ensure consistency and coordination. (2.11)*

Finally, it is asserted that the success of these new reform proposals can
and will only work if NHS professionals play their part in this new partnership

vision. The low trust competitive environment which has developed in recent years needs to be changed if future success is to be achieved. As the White Paper puts it:

> *To succeed in the NHS of the future, NHS Trusts will need to develop and involve their staff. In the past this has not been a high priority. In the New NHS it is – for one simple reason. The health service relies on the commitment and motivation of its staff. That is why there will be a new approach to better valuing staff. (6.27)*

The White Paper thus offers a constructive and positive programme for a new collaborative care approach by the NHS. The Secretary of State is clearly aware of the enormity of the challenge, but refers to his confidence in the support of the public, the dedication of NHS staff, and the backing of the Government.

We will now turn to consider two broad areas which will need attention if a collaborative culture is to be created and the Government's stated policy objectives are to be achieved. These two areas are:

1. Changes needed in structure and organisation.
2. Professional development and support.

CHANGES NEEDED IN STRUCTURE AND ORGANISATION

In this discussion so far it has been argued that while collaboration in care has always been beset with difficulties and barriers, the reforms of recent years have made the situation worse rather than better. In combination, general management, a corporate agenda and the internal health care market structures have made joint working and responsibility sharing more difficult than ever before, and particularly so within the complex and fragmented network of primary health and social care settings. According to Boarden (1997) and Rillands (1997):

> *If integration of provision and shared professional activity are to be hallmarks of future (primary) care . . . existing structures will need to be swept away. Unless this is changed, managers will face a heavy burden in trying to secure interactions between agencies and professional staff.*

Lewis (1997) proposed that a number of fundamental issues, including that of organisational structure and human resources, need to be addressed early on. He lists the areas of immediate concern as:

1. *The parameters of the NHS* – what is, and what is not to be made available universally, and free at the point of need.

2. *The priority of services* – overt decisions made on priorities and rationing.

3. *Sources of funding* – how these are to be found and from where.

4. *Organisational structures* – how these are to be developed, multidisciplinary collaboration encouraged, and how users and informal carers are to be given an enhanced voice in care, planning and delivery.

5. *Use of human resources* – how increasing legitimacy is to be given to collaboration, including authority, development of trust, time and resources for educational support, and development of mechanisms for collaborative working.

Areas 1–3 are of great significance, because clarification of these will demonstrate the political will and commitment to the newly proposed health agenda. Areas 4 and 5, that of organisational structure and use of human resources, very much link together, and are relevant to this discussion.

First we will look at a number of issues around changes in organisational structure. Best & Brazil (1997) express the belief that the NHS needs to move from the centralised corporatist form of governance of recent years to a more collaborative approach, if the Government's policy commitments are to be implemented with some degree of success. They remind us of the potential nature of the challenge which the Government has set itself. As they put it:

> *The Government wants to replace competition with co-operation while moving towards a stake holding NHS characterised by greater equity and inclusivity. [The Government is] prepared to countenance greater local autonomy and variety within a framework of explicit criteria for judging success.*

All in all, Best & Brazil believe that 'these commitments imply a fundamentally new style of governance. They provide a useful diagram setting out in broad statements the differences between yesterday's approach (the corporatist style), and potentially tomorrow's style – that of collaborative management.

The collaborative style of governance as set out below appears to offer an organisational framework which would both require, and indeed trust, professionals to use their particular skills and discretion in care. Implicitly this model values the contributions of people working together at locality levels. However, it will need to be fleshed out in order to ensure the significant inclusion of all interested professional and non-professional participants, and not least the users and their carers. As Nocon (1994) reminds us:

> *The voice of users . . . has been seldom heard, yet if services are to be appropriate and effective, it is essential that users are fully involved in decisions about both service planning and delivery.*

Governance at a glance – how the systems compare

Corporatist

Strong central direction and control exerted through (a) a political line running from the health secretary through regional chairs, to trust and health authority chairs; and (b) a managerial line running from the NHS chief executive through regional directors, to health authority and trust chief executives.

An assumption that the principal roles of the centre are to formulate policy, to vet local plans for implementing policy, and to monitor implementation. The principal role of local management is to implement policy in accordance with agreed plans.

Expectation that local units of management (i.e. health authorities and trusts) will 'sign up' to, endorse and enthusiastically pursue centrally formulated policy.

An emphasis on short term, 'bottom-line' aspects of performance, sometimes to the detriment of less tangible and/or immediate measures.

Relatively closed communication with an emphasis on minimising 'bad news'.

Collaborative

Strong central commitment to agreeing overall corporate goals with stakeholders together with explicit, non-negotiable criteria for judging success. An emphasis on accountability rather than control. Wherever practical, decision making based on the principle of subsidiarity.

An assumption that while the centre sets targets and monitors bottom-line performance, an important role of local management is continually to devise and discover ways of delivering broader corporate goals.

Expectation that inclusivity and cooperation will lead to greater local innovation and energy in pursuit of corporate goals and, as a consequence, deliver more appropriate outcomes.

Bottom-line aspects of performance treated as parameters rather than targets or objectives.

Relatively open communication with an emphasis on transparency and overt public accountability.

(Best & Brazil 1997 Health Service Journal 16 October, p. 25. Reproduced by kind permission of the Editor of the Health Service Journal.)

All in all the specifics of how and in what forms all skills will be harnessed remain to be set out more clearly as the structure and organisation of the NHS develops. It is an uncomfortable reality, but this climate of uncertainty is likely to continue for the foreseeable future. However, what is needed, as soon as is possible, are a structure and a process which will provide legitimacy, resources and time for the development of effective collaboration in care. We now turn to look at the needs of the human resources or individuals involved in providing that care.

PROFESSIONAL DEVELOPMENT AND SUPPORT

According to Lewis (1997) the key resource of the NHS is its staff. Like many others, he notes that their morale is low at a time when the new Government requires their full support and enthusiasm, not least in the collaborative effort. He proposes that staff at all levels should be involved in the debates around the redevelopment of the NHS. By doing this, it may be possible to create a shared vision for the future, and to replace the present low trust environment with one of a more positive perspective. This is not going to happen easily or quickly. It requires the contextual support we have just discussed, together with a change in professional behaviour. As Rodgers (1994) notes:

> *To pursue and achieve interprofessional collaboration, professionals need to value their sense of worth and to relinquish defensiveness.*

As well as developing their own self-esteem and a belief in the value of their professional care contribution, they will need to see evidence of others viewing them in this new light also. Policy makers and authority figures need to demonstrate very clearly that they intend to harness professional nurse skills and knowledge, rather than diminishing and downgrading the level of care they offer – as has often been the case in recent years.

It is evident that for all concerned there is much to be learnt on how to work together more effectively. Continuing education, resources and time need to be made specifically available for the development of skills, and an understanding of the nature of collaboration, to ensure that the mistakes and negative attitudes of the past are addressed, and a new multidisciplinary enthusiasm engendered. At the same time Shipman & Dale (1997) aptly remind us of the need for professionals themselves to recognise the need for collaborative working. They should value and develop a shared understanding of concepts and remits, and acknowledge and act on the need for the development of new ways of collaborative working. Without these attitudes, progress will prove difficult. It will be of little use if professionals and other potential participants continue to be either ambivalent or opposed to the development of shared care approaches.

On a positive note, Gregson, Cartlidge & Bond (1991) remind us of the value of focusing on the concept of collaboration in a meaningful way – the greater the understanding gained, the greater the potential for much improved joint working and a raised standard of care. They refer to the importance of clarifying the differing perceptions, values, expectations, assumptions, behaviours and structures which colour and shape the nature of collaboration in and across health and social care settings.

Biggs (1993) would surely support and approve of such developments. He challenged interprofessional work for its tendency to exclude the users. He argued that it was vital to look at the interface between user and provider in order to refocus attention on new pathways and methods of care provision. A reinvigoration of interest in, and efforts to look at the concept of collaboration in practice would offer the important opportunity he sought.

CONCLUSION

A serious desire to make collaboration work on the part of policy makers, professionals and the public should change dramatically the environment of NHS and community care. In turn, the proposed policy developments for the NHS, all based on collaboration, if well implemented will offer up opportunities to enlarge and to enrich professional care roles, and to improve the standards of care offered. Most important of all is the acknowledgement that complex health needs require an effective multidisciplinary response if a degree of success is to be achieved. Health care professionals including nurses, who claim the centrality of client need as the focus of their care agendas, clearly have much work to do in removing the continuing barriers to effective collaboration. As the Government's public health Green Paper quite aptly reminds us:

Connected problems require joined up solutions. (Cmd 3852 1998)

Good collaborative care would seem to offer a way forward. That said, it remains to be seen whether such an important goal will be achieved in the foreseeable future.

REFERENCES

Audit Commission 1992 Community care: managing the cascade of change. HMSO, London
Barr O 1993 Reap the benefits of a co-operative approach: understanding interdisciplinary teamwork. Professional Nurse 8(7): 473–477
Best G, Brazil R 1997 The personal touch. Health Service Journal 16 October , p 25
Biggs S 1993 User participation and interprofessional collaboration in community care. Journal of Interprofessional Care 7(2): 151–159
Boarden N 1997 Primary care: making connection. Open University Press, Milton Keynes
Command 555 1989 Working for Patients. Department of Health, London
Command 849 1989 Caring for People. Department of Health, London
Command 3425 1996 The National Health Service: a service with ambitions. HMSO, London
Command 3807 1997 The New NHS. Modern. Dependable. Department of Health, London
Command 3852 1998 Our Healthier Nation. Department of Health, London
Fatchett A 1996 A chance for community nurses to shape the agenda. Nursing Times 92(45): 40–42
Flynn R Williams G Pickard S 1997 Markets and networks. Open University, Milton Keynes
Fox A 1974 Beyond contract. Faber & Faber, London
Gregson B, Cartlidge A, Bond J 1991 Interprofessional collaboration in primary care organisations. Occasional Paper 52. The Royal College of Practitioners, London
Griffiths R 1983 The NHS management inquiry. DHSS, London
Hadley R, Clough R 1996 Care in chaos. Cassell, London
Hudson B 1997 Local differences. Health Service Journal 18 September, pp 31–33

Hugman R 1995 Contested territory and community services. In: Soothill K, Mackay L, Webb C (eds) Interprofessional relations in health care. Edward Arnold, London

Hunter D 1997 The challenges of health care restructuring. Nursing Times 93(39): 67–70

Johnston C 1994 Healthcare and social care boundaries. Nursing Times. 90(26): 40–42

Kurtz Z, Nichol R 1992 A case for treatment. Health Service Journal. 16(102): 25

Leathard A 1994 Going interprofessional – working together for health and welfare. Routledge, London

Lewis I 1997 MP Bury South Healthy, Wealthy and Wise. Tribune 7 November.

Marshall M, Preson M, Scott E, Wincott P (eds) 1979 Teamwork for and against: an appraisal of multi-disciplinary practice. British Association of Social Workers, London

Meek H, Pietroni M 1993 Communication in Cancer Care - a reflective learning model using group relations methods. Journal of Interprofessional Care. 7(3): 229–238

NCVO (National Council for Voluntary Organisations) 1986 A stake in planning: joint planning and the voluntary sector. NVCO, London

NHSME (National Health Service Management Executive) 1994 The operation of the NHS internal market. HSG (94)55. NHSME, Leeds

Nocan A 1994 Collaboration in community care in the 1990s. Business Education Publishers, Sunderland, Tyne and Wear

Øvretveit J 1993 Co-ordinating community care. Multi-disciplinary teams and care management. Open University, Milton Keynes

Øvretveit J , Mathias P, Thompson T 1997 Interprofessional working for health and social care. Macmillan, Basingstoke

Owens P, Carrier J 1995 Interprofessional issues in community and primary health care. Macmillan, London

Platt D 1997 In: Healy P. Uneasy bedfellows. Health Service Journal 6 November, pp 10–11

Poulton B, West M 1994 Primary health care team effectiveness: developing a constituency approach. Health and Social Care 2: 77–84

Rillands M 1997 Book review: primary care – Making Connections. Health Service Journal 30 October, p 39

Roberts P, Priest H 1997 Achieving interprofessional working in mental health. Nursing Standard 12(2): 39–41

Rodgers J 1994 Collaboration among health professionals. Nursing Standard 9(6): 25–26

Ross F, Mackenzie A 1996 Nursing in primary health care: policy into practice. Routledge, London

Shipman C, Dale J Dr 1997 Working Together Out of Hours. Journal of Community Nursing 11(7):

Smith R, Gaster L, Harrison L, Martin L, Means R, Thistlewaite P 1993. Working together for better community care. University of Bristol, Bristol

Trevillion S 1995 Competent to collaborate. CAIPE Bulletin 10: 6

Wistow G 1992. Working together in a new policy concept. Health Services Management 88(1): 25–28

8

Learning from the past, looking to the future

The discussions in this book have address two important issues:

1. The developments within the National Health Service (NHS) and their likely form and focus as the NHS moves into the next millennium.
2. The future development of the nursing profession.

In an earlier book I encouraged nurses to be more actively involved in the debate about the future of the NHS in order to shape their own professional destiny (Fatchett 1994). The discussions in this book have built upon that precedent. Hopefully, they will act as a further catalyst for an informed and practical response to what is happening to both the NHS and to the role of nurses. The backcloth to all of the chapters has been that of the Conservative governments' NHS reform programme – the most profound set of changes implemented within the NHS since its inception in 1948. These reforms involved the creation of an internal health care market, the separation of purchaser and provider roles, and the development of an underpinning ethos which is both commercialised and competitive in nature.

In tandem with this major and systematic overhaul of the health service, we have seen what appears to be a redefinition of professional nurse practice. It has been presented as yet another manageable and marketable commodity to be promoted, sold, bought, discredited and even discarded in the business of NHS health care. The root and branch reform of the NHS in the 1980s and 1990s has left no part untouched, be it structure or personnel.

Since the 1997 change of government, this legacy has been passed into the hands of the Labour Government. Consequently, there has been a conscious effort to create a different vision for the NHS, and implicitly within this, for that of the nursing profession also. It is because of this that all nurses have a clear interest in understanding the background to the situation in which they currently find themselves – not least if they aspire to any future role enrichment or full-blown professional status, however defined.

As a consequence, the discussions have revolved around six aspects of NHS change and development, which are central to both professional nurse practice and to the workings of the NHS:

◆ The NHS reforms – past and future.
◆ The focus on health.
◆ The concept of need.
◆ The users of the service.
◆ Professional nurse agendas.
◆ Collaborative care.

Each chapter has highlighted different , but linking issues of importance, set against the backcloth of the internal market reforms, and to the future under a new programme of health reform as set out in the 1997 White Paper 'The New NHS. Modern. Dependable' (Cmd 3807 1997).

Chapter 2: Reforming the National Health Service

This chapter set out to provide a broad backcloth against which all subsequent discussions would be set. The early years of the NHS were outlined, and led into the long period of Conservative health reform and the introduction of the internal health care market. Four successive Conservative Secretaries of State for Health applauded the new approach, seeing within it a modern success story replacing the failure of previous decades. They drew attention to the inefficiencies, the long waiting lists, the inability to listen to the voices of the users, the lack of knowledge about service costs, outcomes and quality achieved. For those responsible for the reforms, the introduction of a market model to the NHS of the 1990s was lauded as an improvement and as a massive achievement of which everyone could be justifiably proud.

There was, inevitably, an alternative view which concentrated upon more negative themes. These centred upon a number of issues: reductions in services, distortions in care provision, a two-tiering of service, widening inequalities in health care provision, greater concern for financial cashflows than meeting need, increasing competitiveness and reductions in standards of care, lack of democratic representation, increased secrecy, difficulty in multidisciplinary collaboration, users' views ignored, staff demoralisation and diminution of professional contributions – to name just a few.

The Government's new health programme in 1997 was supposed to offer a different agenda, one, which it was argued, would begin to address the negativities and perverse outcomes of recent years. Importantly, it appeared to offer the potential for professional nurse development in the future.

Chapter 3: A healthier nation

In this discussion doubts were expressed as to the veracity of the previous governments' stated intention to stimulate a positive health programme for the NHS. The White Paper, 'The Health of the Nation' (Cmd 1986 1992) was viewed as being long on aspiration, but, in fact, making little or no effort to consider the root causes of much ill health such as poverty, unemployment and low economic status. Instead the White Paper emphasised the importance of individual behaviour change and effort. The strategy was not backed up by extra legislation or targets for other government departments. Little extra finance was provided, only encouragement for collaborative action via the loose creation of healthy alliances. For some, it was noted, 'The Health of the Nation' proposals, far from being a new positive health care focused reform, were more to do with reducing the health promotion responsibilities and the role of the NHS, and that of nurse professionals employed within it. By contrast, the Government's Green Paper on public health (Cmd 3852 1998), together with the NHS White Paper (Cmd 3807 1997), seem to provide the possibility of a much broader health agenda. The proposed initiatives could offer a number of important routes for professional nurse contributions in the future. More importantly, the agenda for reducing health inequalities seems constructive, and potentially helpful for the development of the nurse role.

Chapter 4: The concept of need

The assessment of need has been fundamental to NHS activity since its beginning. That said, the concept of need as a measurable notion is 'chameleon like' and adaptable to many different interpretations. As such, the determination of the breadth of health need is very much open to debate.

During the period of the Conservative reforms it has been argued that the concept has been redefined to fit in with the prevailing wish of the then governments, both to reduce and to constrain the parameters of NHS responsibility for care. The language of priority setting, of efficiency and effectiveness, of marketisation and of the pursuit of value for money, has, for example, effectively redirected and reduced professional nurse care activity, not least in response to assessed need.

By contrast, the current Government's proposed health programme could be seen as offering a broader perspective on health and illness, and a new, wider responsibility for NHS concern – not least, that of addressing and reducing health inequalities. For instance, efforts are to be made to ensure the contribution of all government departments to bring about lasting improvements in the public's health. In turn, greater attention is to be given to the expressed views on need of the users, and greater involvement offered to them in the planning and development of relevant services designed to meet the needs of both individuals and communities. Obviously, over time, we will be able to judge the success of these aims.

Chapter 5: Consumer empowerment

In spite of avowals to the contrary, the health reforms of the Conservative governments do not appear to have empowered the consumers. Indeed, it has been argued that far from being *the* powerful players in the internal health care market, patients have been mere pawns in the development of the competitive relationships within and between the purchaser and provider bodies. In a similar vein, consumer power has been reduced, because democratic representation on planning and decision-making bodies has been severely constrained. In turn, the Patient Charters have been seen as nothing more than paper lists of stated intents, lacking financial and legislative backing, and in any case not created by the users themselves. Inequalities in health care, two-tiering of service provision, cancellation of operations, budgets running out, services removed from NHS activity, have been seen in combination as creating a worse, rather than better, deal for the consumers.

The current Government claims that it is refocusing attention on to the users of the service. The White Paper (1997) looks to recreate democratic representation across all of its proposed structural and organisational developments. As with the concept of need, it clearly remains to be seen whether this new determination to make the users central to the care process becomes a reality in the future. There is clearly much road to travel still.

Chapter 6: Nursing and professional development

This chapter discussed the precarious nature of nurse professionalism. It also acknowledged the clear strides in development taken, not least during the recent years. This period has witnessed significant efforts to reduce the power of professional bodies in the health service, and not least that of nursing. Enthusiasm for the development and employment of non-professional carers, skill mixing and redundancy, combined with constant rebuttals as to the professional nature of nurse care, have seen a reduction of support for nursing as a growing profession. As an illustration of this trend, in 1996, proposals were put forward to replace nurse professionals with generic carers (Manchester University 1996). The argument was made that it was more appropriate to employ an individual carer with the specific package of skills needed to satisfy the assessed needs of a client or clients, rather than employing a discipline-bound professional nurse who may not have all the skills required. Very specifically, that particular debate remains open should the present Government wish to explore the possibilities further.

In the meantime, the apparently positive programme offered to nurses within the 1997 White Paper could suggest that this Government has greater faith in the nursing profession than its predecessors. If that is the case, it is incumbent upon all nurses to seize the agendas and to demonstrate the value of their expertise.

Chapter 7: Collaborative care

The promotion of collaboration in care has assumed ever greater importance in recent years. That said, effective and successful collaborative ventures have proved very difficult to achieve. During the period of internal market reform, health and social carers have faced a difficult challenge as they have tried to implement policies, the aims of which often seemed implicitly to be in conflict. On the one hand nurses and other health care workers have been told to collaborate in care, but on the other, the formation of the competitive internal health care market has created an environment not immediately conducive to multiagency collaboration.

The contractual/financial imperatives of the internal market have seemingly created a 'low trust' environment – as theoretically explained by Flynn in 1974. In this situation of low trust, multidisciplinary working is not central to participants' immediate agendas, and as such in practice, is antipathetic to the high trust environment which is believed essential to effective partnerships in care.

The 1997 proposals aim, however, to offer a programme of initiatives (many requiring collaboration in care) which, if implemented, could create and sustain the important high trust relationship needed. To achieve this, experience suggests that a great deal of work needs to be done. Not only does the NHS require a structure and organisation committed to good collaborative working, but a similar commitment is needed from the individuals involved. Professionals must be helped to learn how to work together. More importantly, they have to want to do it, and to have internalised the value of such an activity. In the end, it is only if these issues are addressed effectively that the many collaborative health care agendas proposed by the Government in the White Paper can meet with the success they so clearly need.

LEARNING FROM THE PAST, LOOKING TO THE FUTURE

For many, the highlight of a day at a theme park is to enjoy the latest daredevil ride: the greater the turbulence, the greater the enjoyment. For nurses, life in recent years has been very much like the theme park rollercoaster ride. There is no evidence to suggest that there will be any change to this in the next few years. On the contrary, the best advice for all nurses would be to fasten their seatbelts.

The process of change offers opportunities, even though the quiet life of stability will always appear more seductive. Change, however, there will be: roles will be redefined. For nurses, and their representative organisations, the opportunities will provide a context in which it may be possible to develop a true, new professionalism.

Opportunities, of course, can only be seized through engagement. If there is one theme, indeed plea, from this book, it is that in their own interests nurses have to be engaged in the changes that are taking place, and which will shape their role, and the way in which it interacts with others in society. Passive indifference or sullen opposition are not options: only through constructive engagement can the nurse's role be extended and enhanced, and the profession of nursing achieve greater esteem. After all, the rollercoaster always excites, challenges and reaches its promised destination.

REFERENCES

Command 1986 1992 The health of the Nation. A strategy for health in England. Department of Health, London
Command 3807 1997 The New NHS. Modern. Dependable. Department of Health, London
Command 3852 1998 Our Healthier Nation. Department of Health, London
Fatchett A 1994 Politics. Policy and nursing. Baillière Tindall, London
Manchester University 1996 The future health care workforce. Health Service Management Unit (HSMU), Manchester

Index